A PLUME BOOK

S0-ACY-064

THE CHEERLEADER FITNESS PLAN

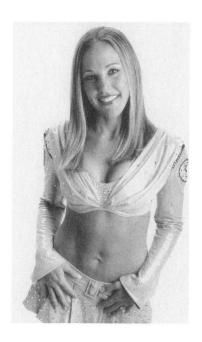

LINDSAY BRIN, C.P.T., B.S.E., is a fitness and nutrition expert and a former NFL cheerleader who has been helping women achieve healthier bodies and minds for nearly fifteen years. Brin was a fitness trainer for the St. Louis Rams Cheerleaders before joining the squad herself in 2005. In addition to her work with the NFL, she is the founder and creator of Moms Into Fitness, of which eleven workout DVD titles can be found in Shopko and Kohl's nationwide, or online at Amazon.com, Target.com, or Walmart.com. Her innovative Moms Into Fitness line is currently the highest-rated pregnancy workout system on the Internet. Brin has been the regional director of seven women's health clubs, holds over ten national certifications, and is the fitness expert for *Fit Pregnancy* and *Mom and Baby* magazines.

She lives in the suburbs of St. Louis with her husband, David, and their baby girl. Visit her website at www.momsintofitness.com or blog at www.lindsaybrin.com.

THE
Cheerleader
FITNESS PLAN

Get Fit and Fabulous
in Just Six Weeks!

Lindsay Brin

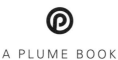

A PLUME BOOK

PLUME
Published by the Penguin Group
Penguin Group (USA) Inc., 375 Hudson Street, New York, New York 10014, U.S.A. • Penguin Group (Canada), 90 Eglinton Avenue East, Suite 700, Toronto, Ontario, Canada M4P 2Y3 (a division of Pearson Penguin Canada Inc.) • Penguin Books Ltd., 80 Strand, London WC2R 0RL, England • Penguin Ireland, 25 St. Stephen's Green, Dublin 2, Ireland (a division of Penguin Books Ltd.) • Penguin Group (Australia), 250 Camberwell Road, Camberwell, Victoria 3124, Australia (a division of Pearson Australia Group Pty. Ltd.) • Penguin Books India Pvt. Ltd., 11 Community Centre, Panchsheel Park, New Delhi—110 017, India • Penguin Group (NZ), 67 Apollo Drive, Rosedale, North Shore 0632, New Zealand (a division of Pearson New Zealand Ltd.) • Penguin Books (South Africa) (Pty.) Ltd., 24 Sturdee Avenue, Rosebank, Johannesburg 2196, South Africa

Penguin Books Ltd., Registered Offices: 80 Strand, London WC2R 0RL, England

First published by Plume, a member of Penguin Group (USA) Inc.

First Printing, January 2010
10   9   8   7   6   5   4   3   2   1

Ⓟ REGISTERED TRADEMARK—MARCA REGISTRADA

LIBRARY OF CONGRESS CATALOGING-IN-PUBLICATION DATA
Brin, Lindsay.
The cheerleader fitness plan : get fit and fabulous in just six weeks! / Lindsay Brin.
p.   cm.
"A Plume book."
ISBN 978-0-452-29575-9 (pbk. : alk. paper)   1. Physical fitness.   2. Cheerleading.   I. Title.
GV481.B74 2009
613.7'045—dc22   2009013436

Printed in the United States of America
Set in Minion
Designed by Victoria Hartman

PUBLISHER'S NOTE
Every effort has been made to ensure that the information contained in this book is complete and accurate. However, neither the publisher nor the author is engaged in rendering professional advice or services to the individual reader. The ideas, procedures, and suggestions contained in this book are not intended as a substitute for consulting with your physician. All matters regarding your health require medical supervision. Neither the author nor the publisher shall be liable or responsible for any loss or damage allegedly arising from any information or suggestion in this book.

To Taylor
for napping in the Baby Björn
for the first eleven weeks of your life
while I wrote this.
And to David
for putting up with my
insanity and loving me.

CONTENTS

Acknowledgments   ix

Introduction   xi

1. How I Became an NFL Cheerleader   1

2. Fitness 101   17

3. Nutrition Essentials   41

4. Eating on the Run   67

5. Exercise Essentials   94

6. A Few Things You Should Know
and a Few Myths You Should Forget   112

7. The Ultimate Six-Week Fitness Plan:
Phase 1—Break Through to New Habits   125

8. The Ultimate Six-Week Fitness Plan:
Phase 2—the "Get into Your Fat-Burning Zone" Workout   175

9. Maintaining Your Weight   218

10. Yoga: Fabulously Flexible   246

Staying Motivated   269

Cheerleader Beauty Tips   271

Quick Reference Guide   279

The Cheerleader Fitness Plan: Goals   291

Food Journal   293

Photo Credits   301

ACKNOWLEDGMENTS

To Scott Mendel, my agent, who started this roller-coaster ride. But gave me the opportunity to write. This book wouldn't have been possible without your guidance.

To Clyde Thomas, my photographer, for making a ten-hour photo shoot easy, and making me look good three months after giving birth!

To Gary Brozek, my ghostwriter, who helped me write this book. Your intelligence and wit are amazing. I'm glad I fit into your schedule of secret agents and sci-fi. And to Dana Demas for putting my proposal together.

To Cherise Fisher, my editor; the first time I spoke with you on the phone you gave me the gift of confidence in being a first-time author. Thank you. And to Jennifer Risser for helping me along.

To Signe Pike, my editor; you were my cheerleader in writing this book and so thoughtful in every aspect of this process. I know if I lived in New York we would have good conversation over lunch! And to Nadia Kashper, I don't know how you do it, but thank you for staying on top of it all!

To Ed and Sharon for loving me and supporting me from the start. Ed, thank you for your illustrations.

To Brent for always being involved and helping make my dreams come true.

To Mom and Dad for your love, faith, and support even when I messed up! Thank you so much for believing in me. I couldn't have done anything in my life without your cheering, making me realize I had the potential to do anything. You've always put your children first, and I hope one day I can be just like you.

Last but not least, to my daughter and husband. David, you give me the support and love that help me follow my dreams. And you make me a better person. Taylor, I love your laugh and your smile. And I love the way you look for me whenever I'm not near. But I'll always be there for you both. I love you!

INTRODUCTION

Welcome! Are you ready for some fitness? This book is filled with insider secrets on how you can live the lifestyle that keeps NFL cheerleaders fit, healthy, and full of energy. You're going to learn a simple, effective plan to look and feel your best that you can practice for years to come. This is a program that's going to change your life—and we're going to have some fun in the process!

Now, I know what you might be thinking. "Me . . . look like an NFL cheerleader?" Or, "I've never danced a day in my life. How can this program help me get in shape?" Well, I'm here to tell you that this program is all about you! Yes, you!

Whether you've fallen off the exercise bandwagon, you're eating all of those foods you know you shouldn't, or you've put on some weight (or all three), this book has found you for a reason. You know how the right people, the ideal job, or other opportunities seem to come into your life at the perfect moment? A healthy lifestyle change is no different. You're holding this book for a reason and I can't wait to share all of the exclusive fitness and nutrition tips, taken straight from my days with the NFL and applied to the everyday woman.

Because real women are what I'm all about. I've spent my career helping women get the bodies they want. Women of every age, every size, and at every life stage. Young women who are just getting started on a fitness program. Women who are preparing to have children. Women who are working to get their bodies back after pregnancy. Women who are years past having children. Women who are gearing up for menopause. Women who are preparing for a life-defining event like a wedding. And women who are simply making a healthy lifestyle change. The bottom line? You don't have to be an NFL cheerleader to put this revolutionary program to work for you. I know you're busy and I know you're (probably) not an NFL cheerleader. So I've made this plan simple to follow for every woman out there.

As they say, life isn't a sprint; it's a marathon. I'm going to teach you how to jump-start your body and your mind in six weeks, and then I'm going to show you how to go the distance with a plan for lifelong wellness. This book isn't about gimmicks. It isn't about fad diets. It isn't about unrealistic exercise plans with fancy equipment. It's about you making a lifestyle change that's going to deliver quick results, but one that is also sustainable for the rest of your life.

I understand that we live in a results-oriented society—we want to see those results and spend as little time as possible getting them. And I know you have a busy life. As a mother, a full-time fitness instructor, and the creative director and vice president of my own company (Moms Into Fitness), I know from personal experience that finding time to get fit and to stay fit is hard! That's why my program is realistic. By spending as few as thirty minutes a day, five days a week, and making better choices about what you eat, you can have the body you've always wanted in as few as six weeks.

I divide that six-week time period into two three-week phases, and provide you with week-by-week instruction in the Ultimate Six-Week Fitness Plan. Included in that is a Nutrition Jump Start with nutritional tips and tricks to help you set goals for yourself, eat smarter, and feel better doing it. Fitness and nutrition go hand in hand, so we'll work on both of them together: all the health experts in the world agree, you can't get fit if you don't monitor what you eat and increase the amount of your daily activity.

Getting rid of excess pounds and reducing the amount of fat we carry on our bodies isn't just about looking good—though that's certainly important—it's also about preventing disease that can shorten our life spans and make the years we have painful. For that reason, I'm going to introduce you to my "Get into Your Fat-Burning Zone" method. Developed especially for busy women who want fast, lasting results, this method takes everything that top-level athletes and coaches know about the benefits of interval training and makes it easy to apply for anyone at any ability level. The exercises I suggest will put you in one of three zones during your workout to maximize your fat burning and conditioning. In combining cardio work with strength training and nutrition, you'll minimize your time (and those targeted zones of fat) spent working out while maximizing results. My workout plan will have you using more muscle groups simultaneously to produce fast results and whole body conditioning.

To give you an idea of how quick and easy some of my fitness recommendations are, I'm going to share with you a few tips about one of the most nagging problems women (and men) complain to me about. No one likes to carry excess weight around their waistline. We have a lot of ways to describe it, and none of them are flattering—a gut, a pooch belly, a spare tire, a beer belly. Whatever you call it, storing excess fat in our stomach region is unsightly and most of us would do anything to get rid of it. Here are a few simple things you can do to get a flatter stomach in one day.

- Drink water! You know this already, so do it. But you've probably heard all kinds of things about how much water to consume. Well, it's simple: eight glasses a day.
- Get rid of the white stuff! That means pasta, potatoes, bread, etc. White flour, starch, and sugar are the biggest enemies in fat wars. This is for one day; I would *never* ask you to eliminate a food group.
- Eat protein and veggies!
- Avoid salty food! Beware the bags and boxes! That's right, prepared foods often contain way too much salt—not to mention other preservatives and chemicals we don't really need.
- Go easy on foods high in fiber if you are not used to eating them; fiber can cause major bloating if added too quickly.
- Exercise! A thirty-minute walk/jog is enough to get you started. Make sure you consume enough water to make up for what you lose during your workout. For a thirty-minute walk you should consume sixteen ounces of water. A rule of thumb for water consumption is eight ounces for every fifteen minutes of activity.

Now, those are simple things you can do for a one-day quick slim-down. But there are a few more concepts we need to cover for you to get a better body in six weeks. Some of this is common sense, but as we all know, common sense is frequently the most uncommon sense of all!

That's also true when it comes to good nutrition. We all know that eating well makes us feel healthier and more energetic. But while we all know that good nutrition can improve our lives, that doesn't mean we always make good decisions when it comes to food. Having tofu in the refrigerator as a kind of decoration won't do you much good. You've got to get in the habit of making the right choices and putting the right foods in your mouth and not just in your refrigerator! My nutrition plan will help you make the better choice among things to eat. Notice I didn't say the *best* choice? That's because frequently we don't always make the best choice. We get down on ourselves then and think, "What difference does it make? I can't eat the best things all the time."

That's totally true and I know it. That's why my nutrition plan is also very realistic. I show you ways to make up for the occasional (and inevitable) slipups. The plan is designed to be one you can follow your whole life. It's not just a diet that you follow for a few weeks until you lose weight. No more ups and downs! Maintaining a healthy weight is so important. That said, I know you want to lose weight, and I'll help you get the instant (and sustainable) results you want.

If you haven't worked out before, don't be intimidated. The exercises I recommend are built to be simple and they require no fancy equipment. You can do them in the privacy of your own home, so you don't have to worry about wearing the latest in designer fitness apparel or footwear. I believe that fitness needs to be both accessible and fun—that's the only way you'll be able to incorporate these changes into your life. Who needs or wants drudgery and negative emotions?

But before we get started, let's step inside the exciting world of the NFL, so I can give you a day-in-the-life of an NFL cheerleader—including why I didn't make the squad my first time around and how this forever changed my approach to fitness. You're going to reap the benefits of my failure!

Just one more thought before we dive in: this book is really just the beginning for you. I'm hoping that instead of simply guiding you for six weeks, these ideas will act as a foundation for you, launching you into a lifetime commitment to yourself and to your health. The mind leads the body. So much of our success in life depends on getting our minds right. And one of the best ways I know to get our minds on the right track is to set some goals.

A couple of years ago at a TurboKick Master Trainer Program, I was asked to make a "To Do" list. This wasn't just any "To Do" list, but a list of the ten things I wanted to accomplish within the next year. Not only did I have a number of things that I'd always wanted to accomplish, I also wanted to be able to check off a few things from my list!

I found this to be a helpful tool in organizing my thoughts and dreams. So, I thought I would share my list, whether you find it obnoxious or uplifting, to help you organize your goals:

1. Spend more time with my husband
2. Become a Master Trainer for TurboKick
3. Clean out the basement
4. Start a family
5. Talk to my brother at least once a week
6. Finish photo albums
7. Become a Rams Cheerleader
8. Grow my prenatal/postnatal fitness program
9. Make others happy, so I can be happy
10. Write a book

Before you turn to the first chapter, I want you to go to the back of the book, on page 291, and write down your ten goals for the year. I'm confident that I'll be able to help you achieve at least one of them. And you know what they say about success, don't you? I have a feeling that once you achieve your fitness goals, you're going to find yourself on a roll and checking all the others off your list as well!

THE CHEERLEADER FITNESS PLAN

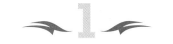

HOW I BECAME AN NFL CHEERLEADER

We're lined up in the tunnel at the Edward Jones Dome, home of the St. Louis Rams. It's finally real. I've been practicing all summer with the squad. I've had my picture taken for the team photo and the swimsuit calendar. I finally realized a goal that I'd set for myself. My dream came true. I'm an NFL cheerleader!

The energy is exhilarating as I stare out into the crowd. Everyone is cheering and the lights are blinding. The announcer's voice is blaring over the loudspeakers, and there is music and commotion unlike anything I've ever heard before. Nothing could have prepared me for my first game day.

We're standing at the edge of the tunnel. It's almost time to run out. As we stand there, ready to run, it's surreal to see the players pumping each other up, getting ready for the game. The intensity is palpable as they keep hitting each other on the shoulder pads shouting, "Let's do this!" And, "Let's go!" They never stop moving. I am mesmerized.

Suddenly, it's time. A wave of insecurities overcomes me. Did I stretch enough? Is my bra tucked away? Do I know all of my routines? Am I going to forget an eight-count when we dance in the end zone?

Go! Before I have the chance to think twice, I forget my worries and I'm smiling from ear to ear as I run onto the field to the wild cheering of the crowd. Adrenaline rushes through me as we form a tunnel of our own to cheer for the players as they run out. My pom-poms are shaking so frantically I think they might fly away. Then we stand for the national anthem and run across the field to take our positions.

I look at my captain. We've spent all summer learning our routines and now it's time to strut our stuff! She calls out a dance and we perform it on cue, perfectly. We're cheering on our Rams and the crowd is going crazy. And the best part is, I've got a front-row seat to a season's worth of football games.

We're cheering "Defense! Defense!" to the crowd. I spot my family who is there to support me. Then we're on offense and we turn toward the players to perform another cheer. I can't take my eyes off the game. When we're back on defense, I look at the JumboTron one time too many and miss a cue. My captain tells me to stop looking up there and stay focused, but sometimes it's so hard to have our backs to the game!

Before I know it, it's halftime. My feet are aching, but I know we're only two hours into the game and my adrenaline is still pumping. We run into our locker room, grab bottles of water and an amazing, dangerous cookie that one of our coaches makes. Contrary to popular belief, cheerleaders don't perform at halftime, unless it's a special occasion. Halftime is our break time! We scramble to brush our hair and apply a quick coat of lipstick before it's back to the field for the final half of the game.

We'll perform twenty sideline cheers tonight, in the end zone and on the field, and five dances. Did I mention we're doing it in boots? By the end of the night, I'm drained beyond anything I've ever experienced. My husband, David, is waiting for me outside the locker room, as he will do after every game. And all I can think about is how I can't wait to do it all over again next week!

Tryouts: If at First You Don't Succeed . . .

My dream to be a cheerleader in front of 65,000 fans started long ago. Not only did I dance and cheer throughout my life, I watched my mother teach aerobics growing up. Yes, she bopped around in her leotard and had fun, but she also changed women's lives while doing it. When I was about eight, I probably went to every class she taught. I stood in the back of the room and imitated everything she did. I just loved watching all the women with smiles on their faces—they were having fun! And they always stayed after class (experiencing that energy high) to laugh and talk up a storm. I don't think she knew it at the time (nor did I) but watching her teach aerobics molded me into who I am today.

We may no longer bee-bop around the room like they did, but I'm here to tell you that fitness can be fun for you. I have a strong background in fitness and have enjoyed doing it every bit of the last fifteen years. Fitness and cheering isn't just what I do, it's a lot of who I am. I started teaching fitness myself in high school and I majored in sports science at college. So, when I met my husband, David, and moved to St. Louis in 2002, I finally had my chance to try out to be a St. Louis Rams Cheerleader!

I decided to train for the tryouts by running a marathon. I thought, what demands a greater level of fitness than a marathon, right? So for the better part of a year, I worked really hard and kept to a rigorous training schedule. I ran most days of the week and, on April 6, 2003, I ran that marathon—all 26.2 miles of it. My time was four hours, fifty-one minutes, and three seconds, about twenty minutes longer than my goal. I was proud of my performance (and sore), but the day I was really training for came about a month later. I walked into the NFL Rams practice arena and the scene was dizzying: the room was filled with hundreds of women who had shown up to fulfill their dreams of becoming NFL cheerleaders, too. There were hordes of media and camera people there to film us throughout the day, watching us practice, dance, succeed, and fail. Although I'd done a lot of fitness work with groups and I was always pumped when teaching a class, I'd never performed for an audience like this before.

Looking around, I also realized pretty quickly that I didn't look the part of an NFL cheerleader. I'd shown up in my aerobics uniform: a gray sports bra, black spankies, tan hose, and my hair in a ponytail. If I'd been prepared, I would have known that I needed to wear my hair down, like the cheerleaders wear it on game day, and I would have put on a much more distinctive outfit. I also barely wore any makeup. I know now, of course, that NFL cheerleaders can't afford to fade into the green field as a result of washed-out makeup! I was trying out to perform in front of 65,000 people, after all.

Regardless, I was determined to give this tryout my all. We learned a routine in the morning developed by the Rams Cheerleaders' choreographer and it was taught to us by an ex–Rams Cheerleader. That afternoon, we tried out in groups of three. Can you say pressure? It was intense to learn a routine and, just a few hours later, dance in front of hundreds of people. We were not only watching each other try out, we also had media and camera people in addition to the panel of judges, which included Rams football players, dance coaches, fitness experts, and TV personalities.

When my group of three was called, I got up, introduced myself, and performed the one-minute routine we'd learned that morning. And then I missed an eight-count. I kept my cool and kept smiling as I stood there trying to remember the choreography, but I could feel my confidence slipping and I knew the judges could see it. I got back on track and finished the routine, but I had a pretty good feeling that of the 250 girls there, I would not be one of the sixty to seventy girls called back for semifinals to create the final squad of twenty-five or thirty.

My fears were confirmed that afternoon when I went home and looked online at the tryout results. Even though I was sure I wouldn't see my name, my heart still sank when I looked at the screen and it wasn't there.

Tryouts Part 2—Practice Makes Perfect!

My training for the next tryouts began on the same day I realized I hadn't made the team. I decided right then and there that next time, I would be far better prepared.

How? By training in a sport-specific paradigm. I quickly learned a valuable lesson that would forever change my approach to fitness. In addition to not doing my homework to look the part, I also hadn't made an effort to get in shape by dancing. My jazz shoes were dusty and I realized with horror that I hadn't touched them for eight years! I wrongly assumed that I'd pick up where I'd left off and that my previous experience would be enough. It wasn't.

I'd run a marathon, but I discovered that doing the same training every day had prepared me for, well, completing a marathon. Running mile after mile did not prepare me to master a one-minute dance routine, and if I couldn't do that, why would anyone put me on the squad? If I wanted to make it as an NFL cheerleader, I needed to start dancing again.

I also realized that I needed to train with interval workouts. An interval workout mixes up the type of exercise you're doing, alternating between fast, strenuous exercises and easier, more low-key exercises. Running on a treadmill for one hour and performing an interval workout for a half hour burn the same amount of calories. It also keeps the mind and body challenged, works more major muscle groups, and targets the heart in a way that a single activity doesn't. This revelation changed the way I got in shape—and it changed the way I teach fitness to this very day. Interval training is the most bang for the least amount of effort. It's fun. It's effective. (And it's what you're going to learn in this book.) I call it the Get into Your Fat-Burning Zone method.

I had spent some time around the Rams Cheerleaders also, gleaning some good insights into what it would take to make the squad. And I had been hired to teach a kickboxing fitness class to the cheerleaders. Talk about an intense interval-type workout—kickboxing kicks butt!

The next time tryouts rolled around, I was far more prepared. I'd been dancing in hip-hop cardio classes. I'd been interval training. I looked and felt better than I ever had before. This time, my dedication showed in my appearance, too. I curled my hair and put on "stage" makeup. I had a hot pink outfit on and though I felt significantly more confident than at my first tryout, I was still pretty self-conscious and incredibly nervous. But this time, I could just feel that things were different. And as it would turn out, luck was on my side. This time, we had two nights to learn the dance routine and two additional days to practice before tryouts. Every day, I was the first girl on the field at the practice arena and the last one to leave. I practiced my heart out and it showed!

When it came time to try out, we watched a group of veteran Rams Cheerleaders dance and show the judges the routine. All veteran cheerleaders are required to try out each year to prove that they still have their physique and that they are still at the top of their game. If they're not, there's always somebody better, and they'll sweep the spot right up. Needless to say, everyone gets into great shape before tryouts, veteran and rookie cheerleaders alike.

As we watched each group of three take their place before the judges, I anxiously awaited my turn. We were the thirty-fifth group, which gave me thirty-four times to practice the routine in my mind by the time I got up there!

When our time finally came, I introduced myself and turned into the starting pose.

The music started and, this time, I nailed it! All of my preparation and targeted training had paid off.

That afternoon, the semifinalists were posted. This time my name was there! Three days later, sixty-five other women and I returned to learn a second routine. This dance was more difficult. NFL cheerleaders perform routines to hip-hop, jazz, country, and other types of music, so being versatile in all different kinds of dance is important. We had individual pictures taken and the next day we had our interviews. I made sure to wear a sophisticated suit jacket and skirt. Finally, we tried out for the last time, in groups of two. We were videotaped for the entire day, through warm-ups of kicks and leaps down the field to the final routine. I knew I'd done my best and I waited to find out the results.

I'll never forget where I was when I learned I was an NFL cheerleader for the St. Louis Rams. We were visiting family and everyone had joined me in the family room to look at the results online. It was Saturday, May 7, 2005, and the results had been promised for 10:00 a.m. Well, by 10:30, they still weren't posted and everyone had lost interest and wandered off. At 11:00, I refreshed the screen and I screamed! Was that really my picture among the 2005–2006 Rams Cheerleaders? Everyone came running into the room and we all celebrated. I had made it—and this book outlines the fitness and nutrition program that got me there.

The Real NFL Cheerleaders

The life of an NFL cheerleader is exciting and very, very busy. We may not be what you think we are. After college, I thought I was too old to be an NFL cheerleader. In reality, NFL cheerleaders are moms, lawyers, dental assistants, teachers, and, yes, some students. My squad's youngest member was nineteen and the oldest member was thirty-four.

The Tuesday after I found out I'd made the team, we had our first meeting. It was great to meet the women that I'd be spending so much time with for the next year. The preseason didn't start until August, but we had practice all summer long to learn the routines that would take us through a four-hour game on the very first game day that made it all so real.

As I mentioned earlier, the body is challenged immensely while cheering a typical game, so preparation is important. A game is the equivalent of a rigorous four-hour workout—in boots. I'd learned a key lesson during tryouts about the difference proper preparation makes, and it would serve me well now that I was on the squad.

We practiced twice a week for three hours all summer and had weekend camps with a very talented NFL choreographer. We needed to learn about twenty-five dance routines and twenty one-minute sideline cheers. This was our goal for the summer: master nearly fifty routines in time for the first preseason game day. We practiced in our "lines," which are groups of six women that remain the same throughout the season. On game days, each line cheers at one corner of the field, rotating every quarter so that the fans get to see every cheerleader. A fifth group is in the arena talking to fans, signing autographs and cheerleader calendars, and welcoming special groups that are visiting.

Lines are determined according to height, so that all the women in a line appear to be the same height. At five feet one and a half inches (I hold on to that half inch!), I was in the group of shorter girls. Every group was expected to become coordinated on the half second, so that kick lines and all of the routines were sharp and in sync. Each line of NFL cheerleaders has a captain. During games, the captain calls off which cheer to do according to the instruction of the coach via an earpiece. During practice, the captains teach their respective lines the routines developed by the choreographer.

Practices were great and long and sweaty. I practiced all of the time at home, too, even videotaping myself so I could be my own judge. It was an amazing whirlwind, and the season hadn't even begun. We received our trademark white boots, as well as our Rams luggage, practice bag, and pom-poms. We were fitted for all of our uniforms—game-day uniforms, practice uniforms, preseason uniforms, charity uniforms, and holiday uniforms. It was all so exciting and I was ecstatic to be a proud member of the team!

Off the Field

Charity work began right away that summer. In addition to supporting the team on the sidelines, NFL cheerleaders are expected to be active members in local and national fund-raising efforts. We were required to do sixteen charity events for the year, which worked out to about one event a week in the summer and one event every other week during game season. We got to know people in the community and also each other for many months before getting on the field.

The events were always a lot of fun. Whether handing out towels at the St. Louis Epilepsy Foundation's Bowl-a-Ram-a or sitting in a booth for the U.S. Coast Guard, as Rams Cheerleaders we were there to raise awareness and create an incentive for people to attend and fund these important causes. My favorite charity was Willows Way, a local St. Louis charity that

MEET ONE OF THE FAMILY

I know it's kind of cliché to say that the people you work with are like family, but in the case of cheerleaders it really is true. On the Rams squad, we even have Big Sisters and Little Sisters. And the lines we practice in become really close-knit. Every now and then throughout the book, I'm going to introduce you to one of the family or an NFL cheerleader from another squad whom I admire.

Tara was a Rams Cheerleader for one year, and is also the mother of a one-year-old child. I spoke with Tara to learn her secrets for looking her best.

LB: How did you mentally and physically prepare for tryouts?

Tara: I ran one to three miles every day, and I did my sit-ups and butt-ups floor workout. And of course, I worked on my dancing technique.

LB: What do you do when you feel bloated? Especially on game day?

Tara: I believe you look how you feel. When I feel bloated or just flabby, I have found that a quick floor workout can really make me feel better. I do a series of sit-ups and butt-ups, and I feel like it really helps tighten things up. In the end, it makes me feel more confident.

LB: What do you find to be the best way to stay in shape?

Tara: I do a little of everything! I have found that doing a variety of exercises helps keep things fun and helps keep you motivated.

LB: Being a mom, how do you fit exercise into your schedule?

Tara: Being a mom is a lot of hard work, but I have found if I continue to exercise, I feel better and in turn, I am a better mom. Because I like to spend time with my baby I try to include him in my exercise. I have a jogging stroller that I use so we both can enjoy a jog in the outdoors. I will turn on my Moms Into Fitness DVDs and do them while he is playing right next to me. I also take him to the gym with me. He enjoys getting in some social time with the other kids.

supports special needs people. I always enjoyed spending time with the participants, as well as their mentors.

All NFL cheerleaders and players do this type of charity work, both locally and nationally. We'd sign autographs, as well as posters, team photos, and the annual St. Louis Rams Cheerleader swimsuit calendar (more on that later!). Some of the events supported charities that Rams players had created or donated to; other events were to raise money for organizations like United Way, local food banks, and other foundations.

Through it all, we were encouraged to look our best and do our best. We were representing not just our team, but also the NFL. Our charity work in the community was as important as our time on the field. If a cheerleader didn't fulfill her charity obligations, she wouldn't make the team the next year. We started our charity work before the preseason and continued the work after game season was over. Because of these charity events, I became incredibly close with many women on the squad.

Of course, we were given some wonderful perks to help us be the best NFL cheerleaders we could be. In addition to getting our hair and makeup done every game day, all of us were given a free gym membership, free tanning, sponsors who did our hair and makeup off the field, and referrals to a dermatologist and dentist who gave us their services at a discount. We were never pressured to lose weight and we weren't required to use any of the services, but most of us certainly took advantage of the perks!

And trust me, you wanted every perk you could get your hands on in preparation for the annual St. Louis Rams Cheerleader calendar shoot, an NFL tradition.

The Swimsuit Calendar

Every year, each NFL team releases a swimsuit calendar of its cheerleaders. Proceeds from its sales go to various local charities. Ours went to a youth foundation to promote literacy in children around the St. Louis area. The swimsuit calendar is a great fund-raising effort that also allows us to interact with fans of all ages. Most fans love to have their calendars signed, and we're happy to oblige.

The photo from my swimsuit shoot still hangs on my refrigerator and motivates me. This picture was taken just after I made the team. I had worked so hard to get on the squad: with dancing, interval training, and great nutrition. The week before the swimsuit shoot, I really stepped up my fitness routine and watched what I was eating, so I looked as good as possible. I followed the simple, safe plan for a flatter stomach in one day that I told you about in the introduction.

We'd started shooting at 4:00 a.m. that day, and it was close to 100 degrees just a few hours later. Of course we had to pretend we weren't hot and still had to look our best! Fortunately, we had hair and makeup people following us around during the shoot. Our coach picked the swimsuits out of several options we brought from home and my husband still takes pride in the fact that my coach picked two bikinis he bought me for our honeymoon! I really felt like a movie star that day. The picture represents me at my best, and it motivates me to reach that ideal again because I know I can get there. We all need something to motivate us when getting in shape, losing weight, or simply staying in shape. I am speaking about something tangible. Something that provides you with motivation on the days you think you can't achieve a new and improved you. Something to keep you going when you're exhausted and can't bring yourself to work out. Something to restore your hope on a day when you've given in to bad food choices.

Everyone's something is different. For some people, positive images are motivating. Maybe you'll tape a picture of yourself at your best to the bathroom mirror, so you see it every day. Or maybe it's a great new dress you're determined to rock before the seasons change. Maybe it's just a note or a favorite quotation that inspires you.

For other people, negative tactics work better! It's nothing to feel bad about and you should do what works for you. Maybe you need a photo of

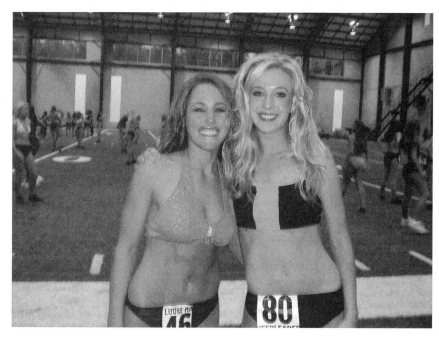

Tryouts, my second time around.

your backside at its worst. Or maybe a lifelike picture of a big blob of fat is taped to the refrigerator to make you think twice before going for the ice cream. Whatever it is, I think it's helpful to have a touchstone for the lifestyle change you're about to make—either the prize that lies just ahead or the life you are leaving behind.

Just so you know I'm in the same boat as you are, during the course of writing this book, I gave birth to a beautiful baby girl. So I'm going to be starting out on my fitness routine to get back to that photo shape again. We'll be going though this experience together!

After my first season as an NFL cheerleader, I continued my charity work, but my husband and I decided to start our family and I didn't try out the next year. Don't get me wrong, there are plenty of NFL cheerleaders who are moms, but being a pregnant cheerleader probably doesn't work! But make no mistake—I will get back my figure, go to dance classes, and try out again! My swimsuit photo still reminds me of my ideal. The program that follows will be my guide back to it. Are you ready to make it yours?

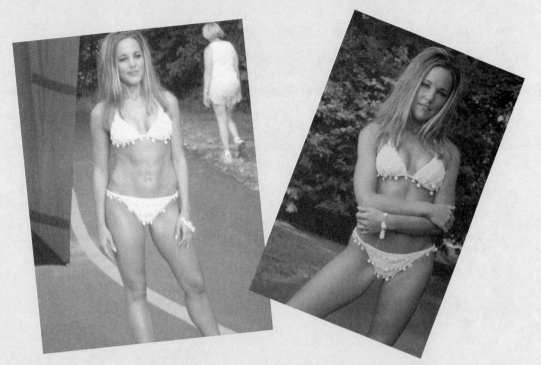

The swimsuit calendar shoot—and the picture that still hangs on my refrigerator.

My official St. Louis Rams Cheerleader calendar photo.

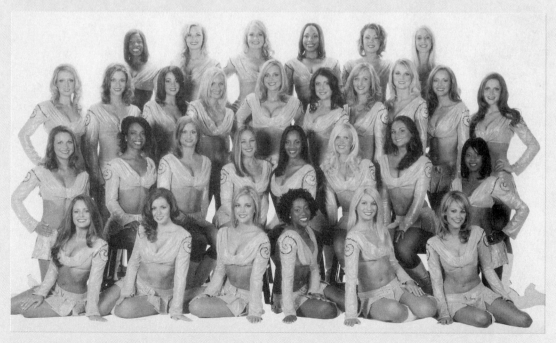

The 2005–2006 Rams Cheerleader poster.

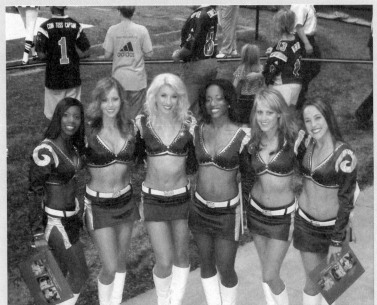

NFL St. Louis Rams
Cheerleader
calendar charity
work.

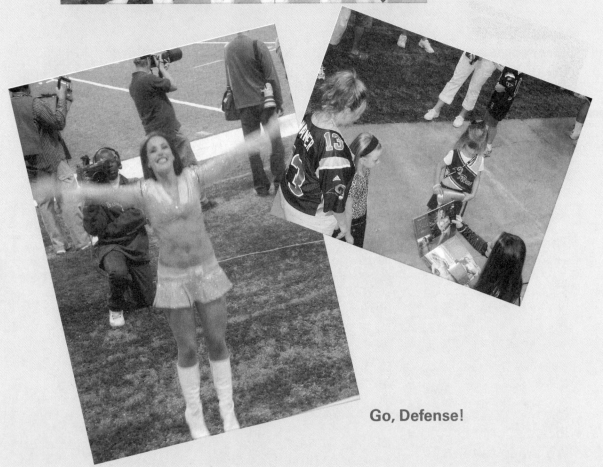

Go, Defense!

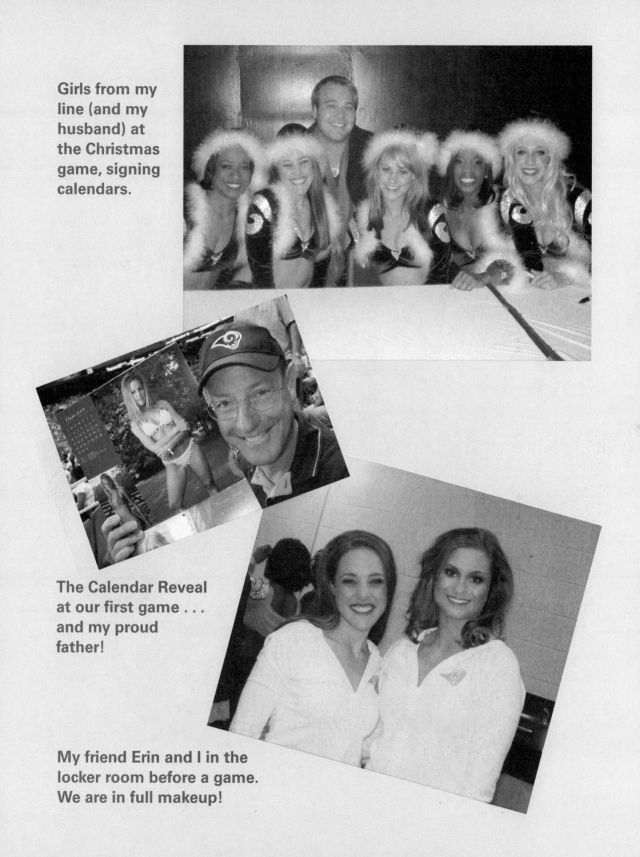

Girls from my line (and my husband) at the Christmas game, signing calendars.

The Calendar Reveal at our first game . . . and my proud father!

My friend Erin and I in the locker room before a game. We are in full makeup!

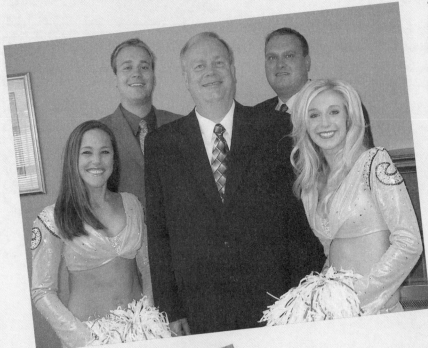

The St. Louis Rams Cheerleader dental sponsor, which happens to be my husband, brother-in-law, and father-in-law!

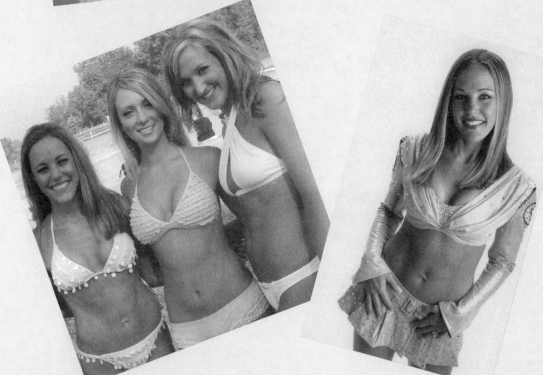

The swimsuit shoot.

My official Rams photo.

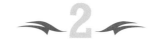

FITNESS 101

I n the last twenty years, we've been told that carbs are good for us and too much red meat is bad and vice versa. We've Tae-Boed and step-classed, done hot yoga and mall-walked. You've probably got a collection of various gadgets like the ThighMaster and some variation of an Abdominizer, and you may have a pair of leg warmers stashed away in some closet. We spent, in 2007 alone, more than $3.5 billion on exercise equipment! And that doesn't even include the $29 billion on sports apparel.

So, as a group, Americans must be looking pretty good, right? Well, I'm not going to make a judgment about our appearance. I can tell you this, though. A few months ago, as I sat down to write this, *NBC News with Brian Williams* broadcast another bit of bad news. According to a story they touted as a hard look at the "diabetes epidemic" sweeping America, they cited figures from the Centers for Disease Control and Prevention claiming that 14.7 million Americans suffer from type 2 diabetes. Worse, they also claimed that another 5 million have the disease but are as yet undiagnosed. The major cause of this disease? Americans' ever-expanding waistlines and the staggering number of overweight and obese citizens in this country. "Overweight" is defined as being up to thirty pounds over "healthy" weight—a sliding standard—and "obese" as being any amount over that.

America's weight gain issues are a harsh reality. By 2010, according to government researchers, 68 million Americans will be obese. That number translates into 40 percent of the population, a 9 percent increase over 2003 figures. This so-called epidemic crosses gender, racial, and ethnic lines. What is most alarming, however, is the number of young people who can either be classified as overweight or obese. For sixteen- to nineteen-year-olds the number of obese individuals doubled in the years between 1980 and 2002. The number of overweight individuals in that same age group increased threefold. While twenty-two years is a long time and you may think those changes are slight given that span of time, let's take a look at even more recent developments:

- From 2000 to 2004 the number of obese females in the sixteen-to-nineteen age range increased from 13.8 percent to 16 percent.
- In that same period and age range, the number of obese males increased from 14 percent to 18.2 percent.

We're not alone in exhibiting this disturbing trend:

- The number of obese individuals in Britain tripled between 1980 and 2002.
- In urban China, the number of obese preschool children increased from 1.5 percent in 1989 to 12.6 percent in 1997.

Consider this: if current trends continue, statistical predictions indicate that only about 10 percent of the population will *not* be obese by the year 2040. While that date sounds far away, it represents a mere generation's passage of time. Ironically, this human inflation is occurring at a time when we have more information than ever about the causes of obesity, have more knowledge about good eating habits, see various diet books sell millions of copies, and are more looks obsessed than at any other point in our history. So what's the problem? Why aren't we able to get fit?

Keeping It Simple

In my mind the answer is simple. Our genetics aren't any different than they were twenty-two years ago. We have just chosen to ignore the simple relationship between calories consumed and calories burned. We focus too much on what we eat (good carbs, bad carbs, high protein, low fat, no fat) and not enough on how much we eat. So toss out the magic diet pills (on which we spend $40 billion a year)—exercise is your magic pill!

We've seen diets based on blood type. We've been instructed to follow the example of the people of Okinawa, the Mediterranean, South Beach, France, and nearly everywhere else. But all those glittery theories shouldn't blind us to the simple truth that unless we burn off the number of calories we consume each day, we will gain weight. If those numbers are in balance (calories consumed = calories burned) then we will maintain our present weight. To lose weight, we have to consume fewer calories than we take in.

The Magic Formula

Calories consumed = calories burned = weight maintenance
Calories burned > calories consumed = weight loss
Calories burned < calories consumed = weight gain

It is just that simple.
It is also just that hard for many of us.

The Psychology of Eating

Many of us have a complicated psychological relationship with food and eating. While I'm incredibly sympathetic and understand that we all bring our own histories to the table with us every time we eat, I'm not here to deal with a lot of those issues. For the purposes of this chapter, we're going to set those issues aside and deal with the facts about food and its relationship to fitness. We're going to take a more scientific and clinical approach to reduce all the extra baggage that comes with eating, as well as our emotional attachments to that act.

So bear with me a bit as we put on our lab coats and eye protection and fire up a few Bunsen burners, because this is important!

As we know, our weight bears a direct relationship to the calories we consume. But how many of us remember what exactly a calorie *is*? A calorie is a unit of measurement. If you know Spanish, the word *calor* means "heat" and the English word "calorie" is derived from the same Latin root. In scientific terms it is equal to the amount of heat necessary to raise one gram of water 1 degree Celsius.

What it really measures, then, is the amount of energy a food contains for your body. Calories power all of the physical processes of the body, giving us the energy to function. A calorie equals one unit of energy, which is why all foods have a caloric content. And when your body burns calories it is burning energy.

So, when you're scanning nutritional labels on a package you're getting the measurement of that food's energy content. Generally, that measure is for one hundred grams of that specific food and its typical serving size. Your body uses the energy contained in the food you eat to fuel the various processes that sustain life and activities beyond mere survival. Any excess calories you take in are stored in the body as fat.

A Few Words on Fat

The good news is that our bodies can convert stored fat into usable energy. The bad news is that when your body needs the energy you have stored in fat throughout your body, it takes it from all those storage areas and not just from one particular place. As much as I'd like to tell you that a particular exercise or bit of nutrition will trigger your body to take the energy it needs from your thighs, that just isn't going to happen.

For most of us, it's usually our trouble spot that is the last to go no matter what technique of weight loss (except surgery) we use. Also keep in mind your body cannot convert fat to muscle; it can only eliminate it by burning it off as a source of energy. The trick then is to get your body working hard enough that it has to go to the last option (fat stores) as an energy source.

How does the Department of Agriculture determine these values? It places food in a device called a bomb calorimeter and burns it. The calorimeter (as you can probably guess) measures the number of calories "burned" or amount of heat given off. Your body isn't as efficient as a bomb calorimeter, so the Department of Agriculture testers just use that data as a framework. Through chemical analysis and an examination of a recipe and its ingredients, they come up with a very close estimate of the number of calories per serving for each of these foods.

It's not an exact science, but since all the calculations are done the same way across the industry, what matters most is that you understand what a calorie is and what it represents—energy to be used in work.

Metabolism

Metabolism is defined as the rate at which you burn calories. Toning exercises will boost your metabolism so you burn more calories at rest, or increase your basal metabolic rate (BMR). And this extra calorie burn helps get rid of stored fat. You will be boosting your metabolism with this fitness plan so get ready to lose fat!

Do you know someone who seems to eat whatever she wants, doesn't seem to exercise at all, and yet doesn't gain a pound? You may have heard someone like that say, "I'm just lucky I guess—I have a good metabolism." They're partially right.

What they *should* say is: "I have a high BMR, which allows me to burn calories while at rest with greater efficiency than many other people." Well, maybe they shouldn't say it like that since they're likely not to get invited out to lunch anymore.

But simply put, your BMR is the amount of energy you need to fuel basic metabolic functions like respiration, digestion, and maintaining core body temperature—in other words, what you need to sustain life. Another way to think of it is that it represents how many calories you burn without any form of exercise. Of course, none of us are likely to sleep twenty-four hours a day, so our BMR alone doesn't provide us with an accurate picture of our basic caloric needs. You can determine your total caloric need based on accepted formulas and how active you are. The number of calories required for physical activities varies, but generally, physical activities require anywhere from 150 to 600 calories per hour. The variables to take into account are how long and how intensely you do the activity, your fitness level, and what activity you're doing.

Simply performing day-to-day activities is not enough to lose weight. Yes, parking farther away from your destination or taking the stairs instead of the elevator will improve your health, especially for somebody who leads a sedentary lifestyle. (I classify these and other activities, like being a mom and chasing after kids, as "bonus calorie burns.")

The range above, 150 to 600, and the number of other variables associated with the BMR, also known as the resting metabolic rate (RMR), seems very inexact—and it is. To combat that inexactitude, below is a formula that you can use to first determine your BMR and then use that figure to determine your total daily caloric needs.

BMR Formula

Women: BMR = 655 + (4.35 × weight in pounds) + (4.7 × height in inches) − (4.7 × age in years)

Men: BMR = 66 + (6.23 × weight in pounds) + (12.7 × height in inches) − (6.8 × age in years)

Here are the calculations for Molly, a thirty-five-year-old woman who is five feet six inches tall and weighs 150 pounds:

655 + (4.35 × 150 pounds) = 1,308

+

(4.7 × 66 inches) = 310

−

(4.7 × 35 years) = 165

_____

1,453

Does that mean that Molly needs to consume 1,453 calories a day to maintain all her metabolic functions? No. We have to do a bit more calculating, especially since you are embarking on a new fitness program. Your BMR tells you how many calories you need to consume to maintain basic body functions. This number is what you need to consume if you were completely sedentary—if you didn't move much at all during the course of a day. Very few people are truly sedentary, but we use that word to describe people who do little or no exercise or walking.

CALORIE-BURNING ESTIMATES

Let's take a look at how many calories you burn if you engage in normal everyday activities. The figures listed below are how many calories you would burn in one continuous hour of performing this activity.

Activity	Calories burned per hour
Pushing a stroller	150
Walking	200
Playing with kids	250
Vigorous house cleaning	250
Lawn mowing	350
Gardening	250

Now, let's look at similar figures for activities that most of us would look on as exercise.

Exercise	Calories burned per hour
Playing football	550
Interval walking	400
Jogging or running	600
Interval jogging	700
Snowboarding	400
Indoor cycling	500
Outdoor bicycling	300–400
Swimming	450
Volleyball	250
Golf (no cart)	250
Basketball	400
Hiking	400
Dancing	500
Kickboxing	500
Hot yoga	500–600
Yoga	300
Pilates (mat work)	300
Interval training	600–700

As you can see from this list, the amount of calories burned while exercising is generally at least double the amount burned in daily activities. That's why exercise is so crucial to weight loss and maintenance. Most of us consume more calories than we should, and it's a lot easier for most of us to add something to our lives (exercise) than it is to take something away (food). That's just human nature. There are a few people out there who like exercise and physical activity (I'm one!), but that's not true of everybody. I do think that once you get past the initial stages of discomfort and unfamiliarity you will, like nearly every one of my clients, develop an appreciation for exercise—especially when you see how quickly it will benefit you.

AN EASIER BMR CALCULATION

Did the section above have your head spinning? I hope not, but if it did, here's a simpler way to estimate your BMR, or how many calories your body burns at rest.

How much do you weigh?   _____
Add a zero to your weight: _____
Add your weight: _____
Total = BMR: _____

For example, if you weigh 160 pounds, you add a zero to that to come up with 1,600. Next, add your weight to that number to get 1,760 calories burned per day (BMR). Keep in mind that this simpler method doesn't accurately account for how active you are.

Also, be aware that most of us don't accurately estimate the number of the calories we consume. We tend to underestimate just how much we take in. Estimates can have a real effect on how successful you are in getting to your ideal weight and shape, so if it's at all possible, do the more strenuous calculations.

Taking a Break from Science

You've earned a bit of a break. Let's take off those lab coats and eye protectors for a while to answer some of the questions that are likely to be bouncing around in your heads.

A FEW WORDS OF CAUTION ABOUT
CALORIES-BURNED CALCULATIONS

In recent years, exercise machines like treadmills have provided users with a tally of the number of calories burned while exercising. These machines usually give inaccurate calorie readings. Even the numbers I gave you above are just estimates. Unless we put you in a human performance laboratory and hook you up to all kinds of sophisticated measuring devices, we can't account for every single calorie you burn during an activity or while exercising. To accurately keep track of your calories burned, we'd have to account for a lot of variables including your BMR, your age, your weight, your level of effort, and so on. These estimates are based on you putting out 100 percent and that's not always possible, nor is it easy to gauge just exactly what 100 percent effort is for every individual.

Another thing to keep in mind is that the more fit you are, the harder and longer you have to work to burn the same amount of calories you did when you were less fit. An out-of-shape or sedentary woman will burn more calories walking than a woman who works out three or four times a week.

I don't know if you've experienced this phenomenon, but I've worked out at health clubs and gyms and seen women come in and do the same routine for the same time and with same level of effort for months on end. They don't vary the intensity of their workout at all, and soon they stop showing up. I'm willing to bet that they get bored and frustrated because they stop seeing the results they did when they first started.

Our bodies are amazingly adaptable things, and they soon figure out a way to perform any activity more efficiently. So, if you are on the elliptical trainer for thirty minutes at level five for months on end, you're not going to have the same calorie burn as you did the first few weeks. Also, keep in mind that your muscles get bored easily. It's hard to work out with the same intensity when doing repetitive stuff over and over again. Which means you must do different exercises to keep your body changing. That's why I'll be changing your fitness program for each week.

Most of you are probably concerned more about how to lose weight than you are about how many calories you should consume to maintain your weight. I get that. So, how do you lose weight? Eliminate 3,500 calories (or one pound) by consuming less calories than BMR and/or exercise enough to burn that amount of calories. Now, if you want the easiest and quickest way to lose weight—do both: eat less and exercise more. But how much less should we eat and how much more should we exercise?

To lose one pound a week, eat 250 fewer calories per day and burn 250 calories a day by exercising.

Once you've figured out your BMR, you know approximately what those target numbers will be for you individually. For Molly, who has a BMR of 1,453 calories, that means she has to consume 1,203 instead. The good news is that once you start exercising, you can boost your metabolism so that you, like your skinny lunch pal, are burning more calories at rest than you did before.

So if you exercise twenty to thirty minutes a day, like jogging or swimming, you will burn an additional 200 to 300 calories. Our bodies are very adaptable, so a little bit of bad news is that once you reach a certain fitness level, you will have to increase the duration and the intensity of your exercise to get the same calorie-burn benefit.

And the most efficient way to reduce body fat (which is really the goal of weight loss programs) is by doing something called interval training. What is interval training? During the time you are exercising, you vary the intensity (how hard you are working) for alternating periods of time.

Body Mass Index

Besides your BMR and your height and weight, you need to consider another component of your body measurements that relates to your level of fitness—your body mass index (BMI). I'm sure that you've seen long and lean individuals who seem to consume endless quantities of food without gaining weight. The truth is that the more lean tissue you have on your body, the higher your BMR is going to be. The opposite is also true—the more fatty tissue on your body, the lower your BMR is going to be. Doesn't seem fair, does it?

So, how do we determine the degree to which we are lean or fatty? (I apologize if it sounds like we're talking about cuts of beef here!)

Obviously, we have more than just lean tissue (muscle) and fatty tissue in our bodies. The chart on page 29 shows the ideal composition of the various components that make up our bodies.

MEET TWO OTHER MEMBERS OF THE NFL FAMILY

Tracee was a cheerleader for the NFL's Kansas City Chiefs for two years. She is now a game and practice coach for the squad. . . and she somehow finds time off the field for her career as a lawyer!

LB: How did you mentally and physically prepare for tryouts?

Tracee: Cheering for three and a half hours on a field with very few breaks is a very strenuous activity, and the coaches are looking for girls that will be up to the physical challenge, so I knew I had to prepare by getting myself into top athletic condition. I spent time in the gym focusing not only on weights for strength, but also cardio for keeping my stamina up throughout the whole tryout. Also, I ate healthfully to ensure I could keep my energy up for the entire tryout process.

My advice to girls is always to mentally prepare for tryouts as well. You need to know exactly what will be expected of you during the tryout process. I suggest going to as many tryout clinics and speaking with former and present cheerleaders as often as possible. The cheerleaders are the best source of information to get yourself prepared for knowing exactly what you are getting ready to do.

You have to be organized long before the actual tryout weekend. Figure out what you are going to wear for the tryout process (some teams are very specific and require different types of clothes, from interview suits to swimsuits), and make sure you prepare all your paperwork—you don't want to miss a single deadline.

LB: Do you keep in shape by dancing? Or do you add fitness to your routine?

Tracee: I love dancing and always want to incorporate it into my fitness routine, but you also have to have other aspects to have a well-rounded healthy fitness regime. I always incorporate weights and cardio into my routine as well and love group classes that have an interval training that includes both.

LB: What are your favorite songs to listen to while working out?

Tracee: "I Like to Move It," "Hey Mickey," "Pump It" (Black Eyed Peas), "Fighter."

LB: You obviously have to keep up your energy. Do you watch what you eat to keep your energy high?

Tracee: You have to watch what you eat. When cheering you have to stay away from foods that will have a high and then crash effect on you. Also, you have to eat a lot of veggies and fruit to stay hydrated. Our stadium is outdoors and when the field is 120 degrees you have to be aware of what you are eating to keep yourself feeling good.

LB: Do you have some thoughts you'd like to share about the importance of women taking care of their health?

Tracee: Fitness and living a healthy lifestyle are very important at any age! You have to treat your body like your most prized possession. You only receive one, so treat it right!

Tristina has been a cheerleader for the NFL's Minnesota Vikings for two years. She is a Pilates and yoga instructor and also coaches a high school dance team, so keeping in shape is a big part of her life.

LB: How did you mentally and physically prepare for tryouts?

Tristina: At the end of last season (football season) I gave myself two weeks off to eat whatever I wanted, and not work out. I think that lasted about four days before I started to feel terrible. So I got back into eating healthy and working out right away. I have a hard time running, so I took cardio classes at the gym about four times a week. Kickboxing, strength/cardio, and spin classes were my favorites, and I also have an elliptical in my house when I couldn't make the drive to the gym. I started eating small portions every two hours and I felt great.

As for preparing mentally, I finally started my scrapbook from the previous season, which made me remember all of the great times that I had on the team. I just had to realize how badly I wanted to be a part of the organization and team again, and the rest fell into place.

LB: Do you keep in shape by dancing? Or do you add fitness to your routine? If so, do you interval train?

Tristina: I don't only keep in shape by dancing. We have a trainer work with us twice a week and I still make it to a spin class or two at the gym. Our trainer puts us through a very intense interval training workout, mixing up sprints and strength exercises, using mostly our body weight. I also run three miles twice a week with my dog, do Pilates, and teach yoga classes. Pilates on the reformer is my new favorite workout for toning and body awareness.

LB: You obviously have to keep up your energy. Do you watch what you eat to keep your energy high?

Tristina: I am a firm believer in never cutting out a certain food category. I think that we need a balance of carbs, proteins, and fats. I also always eat when I am hungry. If I don't eat right away, I know that when I finally do have a meal I will eat too much, and until then I will feel weak. Almonds, bananas, rice cakes, and yogurt are my favorite "go to" snacks. I also have been trying to stay away from caffeine. I know that it will give me an initial burst of energy, but soon I will crash and probably eat something that I shouldn't. I enjoy it on the weekends, and since tall skinny lattes are my favorite drink, I still treat myself to one every so often, but I make it a decaf.

LB: If you are having a bad or "off" day what do you do to get yourself out of the funk? And if it happens on game day how do you get yourself smiling on the field?

Tristina: Feeling depressed or sad about something that is going on in your life outside of cheerleading is difficult to "leave at the door." But it must be done. Finding a close friend to vent to for a few minutes helps me get it all out of my system before I let it ruin the rest of my day. I always talk to my husband or my mom, who usually will be able to put me in a better mood.

On game day, it doesn't take much to get smiling. It is hard not to realize how lucky we are to be dancing and loving what we do in front of 65,000 screaming, loyal Minnesota Vikings fans!

Type of Tissue	Male	Female
Muscle	45 percent	36 percent
Bone	15 percent	12 percent
Total fat	<15 percent is healthy	<27 percent is healthy
Essential fat	3 percent	12 percent
Storage fat	12 percent	15 percent
Other tissue	25 percent	25 percent
Total	100 percent	100 percent

Several different factors can influence your tissue ratio:

- Fitness level and amount of exercise
- Genetics
- Age (generally the younger you are, the more lean body mass you have)
- Nutrition
- Gender (males, on the average, have less body fat than females and more muscle—see why men can eat more!)

So what exactly does your BMI tell you about your body and your fitness level? Along with knowing what your height and weight are separately, it's important to understand the correlation between the two. Simply put, your body mass index is a number that reflects the relationship between your height and weight. Back in the day, we used to calculate BMI by adding five pounds for every inch over five feet. But we now know how inaccurate that formula was.

In recent years, BMI has become an indispensable tool for health-care professionals to use in helping patients understand the link between weight and general health. Calculating your body mass index and knowing your exact percentage of body fat are not the same. However, a high BMI is generally associated with a higher percentage of fat. That's not always the case. Someone who lifts weights or who has a naturally muscular body will have a high BMI, but that number won't be a reflection of a high percentage of body fat. Keep in mind that BMI does not consider the fat-to-muscle ratio. This is one of the known deficiencies of this figure, but we will address in the next section how you can use BMI along with a body fat percentage test to develop a more focused picture of your body's condition.

The federal government has announced guidelines that have created a new definition of a healthy weight. According to the Centers for Disease Control, if you have a body mass index of 18.5 to 24.9 or less you are at a healthy weight. If your reading is under 18.5, you'd be considered underweight. If you determine that your BMI is 25 to 29.9, you would be considered overweight. A BMI over 30 puts you into the obese category. Individuals with a BMI over 25 whose waist is over 40 inches for men, or 35 inches for women, are considered to have a high risk of health problems. The table below summarizes these findings.

Risk of Associated Disease According to BMI and Waist Size			
BMI		Waist less than or equal to 40 in. (men) or 35 in. (women)	Waist greater than 40 in. (men) or 35 in. (women)
18.5 or less	Underweight	—	N/A
18.5–24.9	Normal	—	N/A
25.0–29.9	Overweight	Increased	High
30.0–34.9	Obese	High	Very High
35.0–39.9	Obese	Very High	Very High
40 or greater	Extremely Obese	Extremely High	Extremely High

The additional factor of waist size makes sense, particularly in men because that's where they store their excess fat. For women, the hips and butt are the primary fat storage areas.

The great thing about determining your BMI is that it provides you with an indication of preventable risk. In other words, you can determine how serious your situation is, evaluate your options, and then do something about it. You should have your BMI checked regularly just like blood pressure and cholesterol levels.

There are several ways to figure out your BMI. One is to multiply your weight in pounds by 703. Then divide that result by your height in inches squared.

Here's how we would figure out Molly's BMI:

$$(150 \text{ pounds} \times 703) / 66^2 = 24.20$$
$$\text{or:}$$
$$150 \times 703 = 105,453$$
$$66 \times 66 = 4,356$$
$$105,453 / 4,356 = 24.20$$

Based on the guidelines above, you can see that she is considered to be in the healthy weight category—though just barely.

On the following page is a chart that will help you find your body mass index without having to do the calculations above. Find your height in the top rows—expressed either in inches only or in both feet and inches. Once you've found your height, find where your weight and height intersect. The number in the box is your BMI.

BMI	Height (in)																		
	58	59	60	61	62	63	64	65	66	67	68	69	70	71	72	73	74	75	76
Wgt. (lbs)	4'10"	4'11"	5'0"	5'1"	5'2"	5'3"	5'4"	5'5"	5'6"	5'7"	5'8"	5'9"	5'10"	5'11"	6'0"	6'1"	6'2"	6'3"	6'4"
100	21	20	20	19	18	18	17	17	16	16	15	15	14	14	14	13	13	13	12
105	22	21	21	20	19	19	18	18	17	16	16	16	15	15	14	14	14	13	13
110	23	22	22	21	20	20	19	18	18	17	17	16	16	15	15	15	14	14	13
115	24	23	23	22	21	20	20	19	19	18	18	17	17	16	16	15	15	14	14
120	25	24	23	23	22	21	21	20	19	19	18	18	17	17	16	16	15	15	15
125	26	25	24	24	23	22	22	21	20	20	19	18	18	17	17	17	16	16	15
130	27	26	25	25	24	23	22	22	21	20	20	19	19	18	18	17	17	16	16
135	28	27	26	26	25	24	23	23	22	21	21	20	19	19	18	18	17	17	16
140	29	28	27	27	26	25	24	23	23	22	21	21	20	19	19	18	18	18	17
145	30	29	28	27	27	26	25	24	23	23	22	21	21	20	20	19	19	18	18
150	31	30	29	28	27	27	26	25	24	24	23	22	22	21	20	20	19	19	18
155	32	31	30	29	28	28	27	26	25	24	24	23	22	22	21	20	20	19	19
160	34	32	31	30	29	28	28	27	26	25	24	24	23	22	22	21	21	20	20
165	35	33	32	31	30	29	28	28	27	26	25	24	24	23	22	22	21	21	20
170	36	34	33	32	31	30	29	28	27	27	26	25	24	24	23	22	22	21	21
175	37	35	34	33	32	31	30	29	28	27	27	26	25	24	24	23	23	22	21
180	38	36	35	34	33	32	31	30	29	28	27	27	26	25	24	24	23	23	22
185	39	37	36	35	34	33	32	31	30	29	28	27	27	26	25	24	24	23	23
190	40	38	37	36	35	34	33	32	31	30	29	28	27	27	26	25	24	24	23
195	41	39	38	37	36	35	34	33	32	31	30	29	28	27	27	26	25	24	24
200	42	40	39	38	37	36	34	33	32	31	30	30	29	28	27	26	26	25	24
205	43	41	40	39	38	36	35	34	33	32	31	30	29	29	28	27	26	26	25
210	44	43	41	40	38	37	36	35	34	33	32	31	30	29	29	28	27	26	26
215	45	44	42	41	39	38	37	36	35	34	33	32	31	30	29	28	28	27	26
220	46	45	43	42	40	39	38	37	36	35	34	33	32	31	30	29	28	28	27
225	47	46	44	43	41	40	39	38	36	35	34	33	32	31	31	30	29	28	27
230	48	47	45	44	42	41	40	38	37	36	35	34	33	32	31	30	30	29	28
235	49	48	46	44	43	42	40	39	38	37	36	35	34	33	32	31	30	29	29
240	50	49	47	45	44	43	41	40	39	38	37	36	35	34	33	32	31	30	29
245	51	50	48	46	45	43	42	41	40	38	37	36	35	34	33	32	32	31	30
250	52	51	49	47	46	44	43	42	40	39	38	37	36	35	34	33	32	31	30
255	53	52	50	48	47	45	44	43	41	40	39	38	37	36	35	34	33	32	31
260	54	53	51	49	48	46	45	43	42	41	40	38	37	36	35	34	33	33	32
265	56	54	52	50	49	47	46	44	43	42	40	39	38	37	36	35	34	33	32
270	57	55	53	51	49	48	46	45	44	42	41	40	39	38	37	36	35	34	33
275	58	56	54	52	50	49													

(There are also a number of BMI calculators available on the Internet and you can visit my website for the links to these.)

If your BMI is not in the "healthy" weight range, the next step is to find your target weight. To set your target weight, choose a BMI in the "Healthy Weight" category closest to your current BMI. Once you have determined your healthy BMI, use the following formula to find your target weight.

$$\frac{(\text{target BMI}) \times (\text{height in inches} \times \text{height in inches})}{703} = \text{target weight}$$

FIXING THE BMI PROBLEM

As good and important a calculation as the BMI is, it is not a perfect calculation because it doesn't account for how much muscle or fat you carry on your body. One way to overcome the problem with BMI not accounting for the fat-to-muscle ratio is to determine your waist-to-height ratio.

To figure your waist size, don't rely on the size of pants you wear. For women, measure horizontally at the smallest point of your abdominal width—somewhere between your navel and the top of your hip bones. Take your waist measurement. In this case let's use 28 and divide that number by height in inches—for this example let's use 66:

$$28 / 66 = 0.4$$

Let's say that this person's BMI is greater than 25 (overweight), but since her waist-to-height ratio is lower than 0.5, she is most likely muscular and not fat. How can we make certain that's the case?

Most health-conscious eaters look at a food's label to determine its fat content. How many grams of fat does this frozen pizza contain compared to this Lean Cuisine? If only we had labels on our bodies that let us figure out our body's fat content that easily.

But we all know that muscle is good and fat is bad. So how do we determine the percentage of body fat we're toting around? You can easily get your body fat tested by going to your local gym or health center. They will use a body impedance scale or calipers to determine the amount of body fat you have. The Bod Pod and underwater weighing are the most accurate ways to determine your body fat percentage, but also the most costly and hard to find.

Remember, your BMI is not the percentage of body fat that you carry on your body!

The Truth about Body Composition Measurements

Learning the various ways to measure your level of health and fitness is like a football team scouting an opponent. I know that for most of you, and for most of the clients I work with, you simply want results. You want to lose cellulite, reduce the size of your butt, wear a tank top, look better, have more energy, and generally be healthier. I offer all of these percentages and indexes and formulas to show you the journey I took in my understanding of these concepts for myself, because I do believe that knowing how fit or fat you are is important. Society has put us under a lot of body image pressure, and most of us are pretty competitive, so we do like to know what the score of the game is. We constantly compare ourselves to the ideal images we see on television, in magazines, and walking down the street. And I want you to know where you're starting—fit or fat.

That said, this isn't really a game at all for a lot of people. Serious health complications and risks are associated with weight and percentage of body fat. Knowing exactly where you stand can literally be a lifesaver.

Everyone's body is different in terms of its makeup. Everyone has a different level of comfort and motivation when it comes to the level of specificity and amount of information about weight reduction. But I believe that knowledge is power and the more you know about your body and its particular needs the better off you will be.

Any of these tests will give you some idea of what your body fat percentage is. That figure, along with your BMI, will give you a much better picture of what kind of "shape" your body is in. Also, it can help you in another way—most of us don't want to shed muscle. We would like to get rid of excess fat. By periodically undergoing these assessments as you move through any kind of weight loss or fitness program, you are going to benefit greatly from accurate feedback.

For this program I recommend you measure yourself every few weeks (use a measuring tape to measure the largest circumference of your arm, chest, one inch above your belly button, one inch below your belly button, hips, and a thigh). Use this as a guideline of weight loss and motivation. And for fun get your body fat percentage tested before you start and at the end of this six-week program.

We're all concerned about fat, so what are the relative ranges of body fat on the human body?

Women

10–12 percent	essential
14–20 percent	healthy range for athletes
21–24 percent	fit
25–31 percent	acceptable
>31 percent	obese

Men

2–4 percent	essential
6–13 percent	healthy range for athletes
14–17 percent	fit
18–25 percent	acceptable
>25 percent	obese

I want to remind you again that "normal" is a very slippery term when talking about fat and weight. Depending upon your age, body type, and other health issues you are dealing with—as well as your level of physical activity—your weight, BMR, BMI, and body fat composition are in some cases not going to fall uniformly into a consistent category.

That's where the tests of body fat percentage come in handy: in combination, all three of these indicators—weight, BMI, and body composition—can provide you with the clearest picture of the total physical makeup of your body. Your BMR along with other blood chemistry analyses (good and bad cholesterol) and heart rate and blood pressure can measure what state your body's internal organs and processes are in. Having this complete picture of your overall condition is an important part of any fitness or weight loss program. It's extremely important that you check with a doctor before beginning any exercise routine. I say that not just for your safety but as a motivational tool. Knowing where you are at the beginning will help you set some realistic goals for yourself.

Okay, so throughout this chapter I've made a number of references to gender differences in terms of fat storage, body composition, etc. Let's get this out of the way. It just ain't fair. Men have more lean tissue than women do. Nothing we can do about that advantage. It's also true that it is easier for men to lose weight. Why? Because that lean tissue responds well to toning exercise and enables men to burn more calories while at rest. Men's bodies provide them with a kind of weight loss head start, but remember, ladies, women not only live longer on average than men do, but we excel at cardiovascular endurance. Have you ever been in an aerobics class where the men get red in the face or leave ten minutes into the class? They may have more muscle mass, but we kick their butts in cardiovascular endurance! And maybe that's why aerobics classes seem to be made up of mostly women . . . hmmm.

Since "fit" is in the eye of the beholder, let's talk about another genetic disadvantage that women have to overcome. Cellulite.

I mentioned before all the money we spend on exercise equipment. What about the lengths we'll go to rid ourselves of cottage cheese thighs or a dimpled tushy!

With all the misconceptions about getting rid of cellulite—creams, dissolves, wraps, etc.—I want to clear up a few things for you. First and foremost cellulite is just plain old fat. And the only way to get rid of it without surgery is through nutrition and exercise, mostly exercise.

I could stop here and say that's all you need to know, but I will go a little further: the more muscle you have, the smoother look you can get. But there is one major reason some fit women can still have cellulite. Women have connective tissue that separates fat cells into compartments, and these compartments look like a honeycomb. This fat then has a chance to protrude and create the cottage cheese effect, through the honeycomb. Your genetics determine where and how many fat cells you have, but through exercise you can minimize the appearance of cellulite.

So why don't men seem to have cellulite like women? The answer lies in male genetics. Instead of the honeycomb connective tissue they tend to have horizontal patterns, leaving less room for fat to protrude.

So how do you minimize the look of cellulite? First, exercise regularly to decrease the odds of developing cellulite. *But*, if you already have cellulite you can diminish the dimpled look with regular exercise. You should do a combination of toning and cardio. The best (and easiest) way to achieve this is through interval training. Follow short spurts of cardio with a few sets of toning. Overall toning is the most important component of losing the dimples! And muscle boosts your metabolism, which helps you burn the fat!

Keep in mind nutritional decisions are very important in fat loss and cellulite minimization.

Now, you can't do anything about the past or your genetics, but you can do a lot about your future. I'll talk about this a lot more in the pages ahead, but the best thing you can do is begin a consistent workout program three to five times per week with toning and cardio (which, if you're going to do the zone interval workout I recommend, you already will be), and you will see significant cellulite reduction within six to eight weeks.

A few words about those creams, wraps, and surgery to reduce cellulite. No cream applied to the skin can penetrate and rearrange the fat cells beneath the surface. You can compress fat, and this is why some methods seem to work—temporarily. Wraps only work for up to about three days. Liposuction permanently removes fat cells, but if more than 10 percent of the weight is gained back, new fat cells will develop. And old fat cells simply get bigger.

As we women get older, our skin gets a little thinner. So even a little bit of cellulite will show through. Combine that with our metabolism getting a little slower as we age, and our fat production increases. Avoid this vicious cycle and get on an exercise cycle! Seriously, take the opportunity to be proactive and prevent excess cellulite!

One pound of lean muscle versus one pound of fatty tissue.

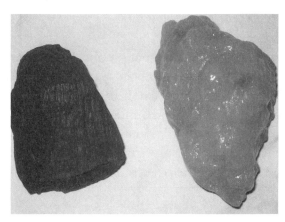

As the illustration on the previous page shows, fat tissue isn't exactly attractive. Fat is rigid and ugly, while muscle is smooth and takes up less space. Fat actually makes your waistline bigger by just being fat, as it takes up more space than muscle.

Getting Fit

Have you heard "if you eat this way, you'll lose tummy fat" or "if you do this exercise, you'll lose weight in your hips"? I hate to tell you, but it's not true. There isn't a single exercise or food that will cause your body to remove fat from one place or another. Your body's genetics determine where to remove fat and where to gain fat. So if your mom tends to gain weight in her hips, your genetics might make you gain weight in your hips, but lose in your tummy. We all have genetics. The *key* is what we do with our genetics to better ourselves!

Now you *can* improve and tone problem areas with certain exercises. If you exercise and eat right you will lose fat from all over your body, including your problem areas.

Okay, so far in this chapter we've talked a lot about where you are today. What about how we get to that ideal self we've visualized? How do we get there? Exercise is one part of making that vision a reality. But nutrition is also part of the battle to lose weight. We're going to talk a lot about various exercises you can do to improve your fitness level in the chapters that follow. *To get your body to react and lose weight you must do a variety of exercises.* Staying on the treadmill for sixty minutes every time will mean eventually you would have to do it twice as long to see results. Using interval training will get you where you want to be *fast*! And even better, it will eliminate the plateaus altogether.

I'll give you a whole lot more about specific fitness recommendations later on, but for now, put down this book and go for a twenty- to thirty-minute walk! When you get back, I'll be here cheering you on for achieving a first down in your march toward a fitness touchdown. If you've had a problem sticking to a fitness routine in the past, you will find this fun and motivating. Especially when you see results the first week. But you must be consistent to see results—both in exercise and in nutrition.

So what does an NFL cheerleader do if she is feeling bloated on game day? Or if she is simply having a bad day? Here are some cheerleaders' secrets for fitting into those two-piece uniforms:

April, a three-year Oakland Raiderette veteran and mom:

I really believe in the power of exercise. When I'm having an off day, doing some type of aerobic activity, especially dancing, always improves my mood. Sometimes when I come to rehearsal, I feel tired but once we start to warm up and break a sweat, I feel so energized. I also feed off the energy of my teammates during rehearsals.

Ashley, a three-year Houston Texans veteran:

If I ever feel bloated, what helps give me confidence to get into my Texans uniform is putting on my pantyhose. The pantyhose really helps to suck you in and give you that finished look all the way around. To keep from getting bloated, however, I try not to eat unhealthy foods that often cause it.

If ever I'm having an off day, what makes me feel better is getting a good night's rest and coming back the next day and killing it at practice or on the field!

Erin, a three-year St. Louis Rams veteran:

Feeling bloated on game day is very distracting for me. If I feel bloated, I stay away from milk or anything carbonated, sugary, or salty. Water is definitely the best option for me, and I try to sip water throughout the day. I also eat lighter meals with vegetables and proteins. Doing a short ab workout can help minimize feelings of bloating for me by tightening the ab muscles.

I like to think that I'm a very positive person; however, like everyone else on this earth I, too, have off days. I try my absolute best to take a step back, take a deep breath, and recognize that things might not be going exactly right, but all I can do is not let it get me down or further distress me, and do all I can to correct it. I try to set those feelings aside and concentrate on the task at hand. On game day, I just realize that I'm so grateful to be out on the field and lucky to be dancing and performing for fans of a sport I love, with twenty-four other women who are all amazing people. I really try and appreciate the moment in all its excitement and this motivates me to continue doing the best I can.

Brianna, a two-year Minnesota Vikings veteran and mom:

If I have an off day I can usually relate it back to either my diet or my workout. If I skipped the gym, or put something in my body that doesn't really belong there, I can feel it mentally and physically. If it is a day where I have no practice, to snap out of it I will go for a run. That always helps make me feel better. If it is game day and I wake up feeling "off," I suck it up, get to the dome, and work out in the morning with my team. Surrounding myself with my best friends and an opportunity of a lifetime is all I need to snap out of my rut. Thinking before my actions in regards to being fit keeps me on my toes and prevents off days.

Brooke, a four-year Arizona Cardinals veteran:

I try to drink a lot of water. Even though you'd think it would cause you to feel more bloated, it actually has the reverse effect. I also try not to eat food with sodium, so I stick to oatmeal, brown rice, and fruits and veggies.

My energy is directly related to my diet. I try to eat well, cutting back on carbs in the afternoons and evenings. But nights before a game I always eat a lot of carbs because I'll need them on the field the next day. I try to eat well six days a week and give myself a "rewards" day where I can eat anything I am craving. I eat a lot of oatmeal, fruit and veggies, protein shakes, and chicken. I also stay away from soda and drink green tea and Emergen-C. I try to track what I eat through a food journal so I know how much I've really had for the day.

NUTRITION ESSENTIALS

Okay, take a deep breath. Get ready for it, here it comes!

The good news is I don't believe in the word "diet." You get to eat! But you need to know the basics of nutrition to understand how it all works. In chapter 2, I suggested that learning about the various ways to measure your level of fitness was like a football team scouting an opponent. NFL teams do look at statistics and they are important. Ask any real fan of the NFL about their team's numbers, and they will give you a long list of facts and figures. You may think that's all just a bunch of trivia, but the truth is that those numbers are a reflection of real-world performance out on the field.

Well, as cheerleaders, we weren't put through the same kind of rigorous number crunching as the players were, but we did have to constantly self-check and measure ourselves against standards that our coaches had set up. More important, we had to measure up to our expectations of what we thought we were capable of. Unlike the St. Louis Rams players, we didn't have someone videotaping our every move on the field, and we didn't have to sit in long "tape sessions" going over, play by play, the last game we cheered at, but we did do a lot of that individually. I know that after a game, I'd replay in my mind how I did during time-outs, at halftime, etc. You constantly have to monitor your own performance to better understand your strengths and weaknesses. As someone told me once, good performers practice what they are good at, but great performers practice what they're good at and what they're not so good at.

In this chapter, we're going to look at how we eat and exercise. Then we're going to learn some game plans to help you tackle your upcoming opponents.

Because you can achieve fat loss without "dieting." Eating healthy is a lifestyle change, and you will learn the fundamentals of staying lean and fit using good nutrition and the menu secrets that keep NFL cheerleaders looking great year-round (but especially before the annual swimsuit calendar shoot!).

I want you to think of diet and exercise (nutrition and fitness) as two halves of the same team. Nutrition is like the defensive team in football. Your goal is to prevent too much of the wrong things from ending up in the end zone of your mouth. On the flip side, fitness is like a football team's offense. Instead of reacting against what your body is telling you it wants, you will be taking charge of the ball and proactively moving yourself forward to score. Your ultimate goal will to be get into the end zone of calorie- and fat-burning activity. If you overeat every day you simply cannot lose weight. A registered dietitian once told me that we don't notice a reduction of 20 percent of our usual food intake, but we would notice 30 percent. So even if you don't do anything else I say, follow this and you should lose weight! Try it today—it's a mental game and it's as easy as eating on a smaller plate.

Before we get to the heart of the matter, let's put a few things about diet and exercise programs into perspective:

- Society makes it difficult to eat healthy *but*—we choose rightly and wrongly what we want and need to eat.
- Ninety percent of all diets fail in the first three weeks, when our faith is most sorely tested.
- Most exercise/fitness programs fail in the first three weeks.

What do you notice about two out of three of those statements? The magic number seems to be twenty-one days. That's right, it takes that long to break old bad habits and break in new better habits. If you can get through that twenty-one-day period (quick: how many touchdowns and extra points does it take to reach twenty-one points?), you've gone a long way toward successfully executing your game plan. That's why I have designed my program into a six-week period. You have two three-week phases. Once you get over that initial three-week hump, we turn things up a notch.

Think of this initial three-week period like the preseason training camps the players and cheerleaders have to go through. While what we did to get in shape and to sharpen our skills in the preseason wasn't fun, it was necessary. Same for the players.

Dance camp is long and physically demanding, and three-hour practices on the field in the dead heat of summer are exhausting! But later on, we get to bask in the glory of Sunday afternoons, cheering on our favorite football players in front of thousands of adoring fans. You may not have the opportunity to strut your stuff in front of that many fans, but you can enjoy the same sense of satisfaction in your accomplishment. Those first three weeks will be tough, but stick it out and the rewards await you.

I remember how anxious I was about having to appear in the swimsuit calendar. I'm as conscious of my body's imperfections as the next person, and being surrounded by so many gorgeous and fit women didn't make it any easier. I knew that if I wanted to look good and feel good about myself, I was really going to have to apply myself during the workouts leading up to the swimsuit calendar photo shoot. I gave it my all and I have to say it was worth it!

It feels like such an accomplishment the moment the coach flips through the calendar for the first time as the whole squad watches, and you see yourself and think, "Wow! That's me!" We all carry around images of ourselves in our minds. The before and after difference was pretty startling and impressive. The after was certainly gratifying!

Three Weeks and You're Out?

Does that mean that once you hit the three-week mark of any diet and exercise program that you're home free? No. It means that things will get easier from that point forward. I've told you about the excitement of cheering in the first game of the season, but as the year went on, some of the women on the team found it harder and harder to really get up for every game. I never got to the point that I viewed being an NFL cheerleader as just another day at the office, but I can see how that could easily happen.

I've also seen this happen with my clients and in my own workouts. After the novelty wears off of doing something new and exciting, you will have to avoid what some call diet (or exercise) fatigue. That's the point when temptation and boredom team up on a blitz. As the name suggests, you get tired of the new same old, same old. But with this program you'll move through different stages, do a variety of exercises to avoid falling into that midseason rut.

Keeping Track

Studies on obesity conducted over the last forty years have shown that most people who successfully lose weight keep a log of everything they eat. Keeping a daily food diary is important—especially in that critical first three-week period. Not monitoring yourself is like a team losing track of what down it is, or what cheer out of thirty routines will come next. As a cheerleader, nothing would be as embarrassing as cheering for a score against your own team. Paying attention and keeping track are critical. As I said previously, knowledge and information are important equipment in the fitness game you are playing with yourself.

After all, our very DNA knows that if we don't eat enough, we will not survive. So when your DNA receives a signal that there is a potential starvation situation, it will trigger a response to seek out food. Meanwhile your body will hold on to those fat stores for dear life when it thinks it's going to be starved. Your body thinks long term and it will do everything it can to hang on to what it thinks is its last precious energy resource—fat. In most people DNA will win the battle against their willpower.

One of the ways to fortify your willpower is to become as conscious as you possibly can be about what you eat. That's where a food log comes in handy. You can take a pocket notebook with you during your own three-week "preseason training camp" (Phase 1 of the fitness plan) and write down everything you eat and drink. You can easily break down your consumption into three sections: morning, afternoon, and night. These three sections correspond to the three main meals we normally eat in a day. You *are* eating at least three main meals per day, aren't you? Skipping meals isn't a sound dietary principle. Most people who "skip" one meal (typically one of the first two of the day) end up firmly planting themselves in front of an even more calorie-rich meal later. Either that or they graze all day, nibbling and sampling at a rate that far exceeds what they should be consuming, or what they would be consuming if they ate a regular meal at a regular time. To combat this kind of skipping and grazing nonsense, I will provide you with specific meal plans in the chapters ahead.

For that reason, I recommend noting the times you eat each thing as well as what you eat. At the end of the day or at the end of the week, look back at your food log and see if you can identify any of your "opponent's" tendencies. Are you an "after-eight" snacker? Do you manage to control your appetite and then succumb to temptation once the sun goes down and the TV comes on? Do you find yourself hunting for a sugar fix at

Time	Food Item	Quantity	Average Calorie Content
Morning			
8:00	Starbucks medium (grande) latte with whole milk	16 oz.	220
8:15	Cinnamon raisin bagel	1	300
10:30	Snickers bar	1 3.7-oz. bar	280
10:45	Water	6 oz.	0
11:00	Pepsi	1 12-oz. can	150
Afternoon			
12:30	Chicken salad sandwich	1	600
12:30	Fig Newtons	4 cookies	56 × 4 = 224
12:30	Water	12 oz.	0
3:30	Potato chips	4 oz.	310
Night			
6:30	New York strip steak	6 oz.	578
6:30	Baked potato (white)	1 medium, 4.8 oz.	130
6:30	Butter	3 pats	3 × 36 = 108
6:30	Green beans	1 cup	35
9:00	Vanilla ice cream	½ cup	300
Total			3,235

three o'clock in the afternoon? Are you fooling yourself into believing that a soft drink is just a beverage and doesn't count toward your calorie total? No matter what your tendencies are, you will benefit from learning them, and if necessary correcting them, by keeping a food log.

Here's a sample one-day entry from our friend Molly's food diary.

Notice that Molly also included the number of calories she consumed. We'll get back to that point in a minute and I've got some suggestions on how to get those numbers easily. For now, let's just look to see if there are any outstanding tendencies we can identify. She does a good job of eating her three meals and so far the only glaring omission I notice is that she doesn't drink enough water (more on water consumption and its fat-reducing capabilities later).

Remember from chapter 2 that Molly's BMR is 1,453. So if her food journal looks like this most days, unless she is working out more than four hours a day, she will be gaining weight. You will also notice she eats few veggies and no fruit, what I consider wholesome foods. While I would love to tell you to eat only wholesome foods, I know that won't happen for all of you.

The great thing about my program is it doesn't matter if you don't make that change. You can simply modify how much of what you eat so that you reduce the number of calories you currently consume. Eating what you love but less of it is a good choice. But the better choice is to change those eating habits completely.

Setting Goals: Working Toward the Touchdown

As is true with most things in life, deciding to get fit will be easier if you have a specific goal in mind. It's far easier to stray from a path when you don't have a clearly identified end result in mind. In chapter 2, I presented a number of indexes that you can use, and there are others—by dress size, waist size, etc.—you could also use as indicators of your fitness level. (For our intents and purposes we're just going to measure ourselves.)

One of my short-term appearance goals was to look fab for the calendar shoot. That was a short-term goal for me because I was already in the best shape of my life. The week before the shoot I zeroed in on my workouts and calories. I want you to set a short-term goal now.

Do you want to look fab in a bikini in three weeks at the lake party? Do you want to drop a dress size by the time of your friend's upcoming wedding? Whatever it is, write it down. The more specific your goal the better. Also write your long-term goal, maybe six months from now. I know your six-week goal is to look and feel better. And with this program you can easily take off ten to fifteen pounds!

In order to know what "better" really means and to track your improvement, you have to record where you start. Just like when we cheerleaders learned a brand-new dance, we knew we could only get better. Our line started off with arms out of place and formations off. But we got better and came together as a line. Just as a football team's choice of plays to be run will be dictated by where they are on the field, depending upon how much territory you want to cover, your goal will also vary.

You should record your measurements—the largest circumference of your arm, chest, one inch above your belly button, one inch below your belly button, hips, and a thigh—every week in the front of your journal.

LONG-TERM GOALS

Remember when I had you write down your ten goals for the year? Well, those could be short-term or long-term goals, but the point was to get you thinking further into the future. If you could check off the majority of those things on your major To Do list, you'd definitely win the game. Think of each of those accomplishments as a smaller victory—a touchdown worthy of being celebrated.

When I set out to be an NFL cheerleader, I didn't get there right away. In some ways, I'm glad that I had to work as hard as I did and that victory didn't come so easily. It made the victory taste that much sweeter, and it also made me realize how I had to focus and set my priorities and take small steps to get across that goal line.

With your fitness and nutrition goals, you'll be doing the same thing.

SHORT-TERM GOALS

Getting to that target weight and BMI is like scoring a touchdown. In most cases, teams have to run a series of plays in order to do that. In addition to your ultimate goal, you should set yourself some preliminary goals. It's hard to think about losing forty-five pounds. None of us have a play in our playbook that will produce that kind of result instantly. None of us are so talented that we can go from sitting at home one day to making it through the series of tryouts to get on an NFL cheerleading squad the next. So we have to think about putting together a sustained drive, with first down after first down, eventually producing the desired outcome—a touchdown!

This is important psychologically—we all need rewards. That's what a cheerleader does for a team—provides them with little rewards and encouragement along the way. In the example above, setting a realistic, attainable (but still tough) three-week goal is essential. At the end of that first three weeks, it would be reasonably challenging for you to have shed five pounds.

At the end of our six-week program you should find that ten to fifteen pounds will have melted away. We will go about losing the weight the right way so it stays off. Besides, losing five pounds in one week is all water weight. It's impossible to lose five pounds of fat in one week. Now, five pounds of fat in three weeks is very possible using our zone interval workout along with the Nutrition Jump Start. To be realistic and have attainable goals you cannot just stay at home. I realize you will be eating out, going out, and doing things you enjoy doing. I *will* ask you to eliminate alcohol for the first three weeks but you can eat out and eat what you want for the most part.

Keeping Score

Obviously, to figure out how you're doing, you're going to have to do weigh-ins periodically. You'll also have to see how your new weight affects your BMI. This is where your food diary comes in. As a part of your three-week preseason (Phase 1), you are to track everything you eat each day. Whether it is a single M&M candy or an entire pepperoni pizza (with all those veggies you are going to add—ha-ha, yes, you will) or any beverage (including water), you are to write down what you eat and drink and how much of it you eat and drink. If possible, using the nutrition information on the packaging, track the number of calories you've consumed. You can also use one of the many online nutritional guides to help you determine the number of calories typically contained in specific foods.

Two invaluable websites you may wish to consult for information regarding the calorie content of various foods are www.nutritiondata.com

and www.thecaloriecounter.com. Not only do they provide you with the total number of calories, they also provide you with an analysis of that particular food's ingredients; its good and bad points; a caloric ratio pyramid, which shows how many calories come from each of its component micronutrients; the fullness factor; and a number of other helpful bits of information. Perhaps best of all, it also includes data on the vast majority of fast-food franchise menu offerings. This is an invaluable tool for you to utilize as you complete your food diary.

Our Nutrition Jump Start plan, which we will explain later, offers an easier method than counting calories. So, while we do need to talk about the importance of calorie counting, we also need to expand on what the Jump Start plan includes—how much to eat of each food group, with visuals (using your hand size for comparison). Believe it or not, all this science is not an exact science . . . and who wants to count calories all day?

"Normal" Calorie Consumption

So, okay, you're keeping track of what you eat and how many calories you consume. Now let's turn to another question. How many calories should you be consuming? According to the U.S. Department of Agriculture's most recent guidelines, males aged thirty-one to fifty should consume 2,000 calories per day. For women in that same age range, the recommended intake is 1,800. And the National Institute of Health recommends that women seeking to lose weight should consume somewhere between 1,000 and 1,200 calories per day.

Remember when we were calculating basal metabolic rates? Now is when you need to do this calculation for yourself to get an even better idea of the difference between what you *should be* consuming and what you *are* consuming. To refresh your memory, grab a calculator and go to page 22 (or page 24 for the simpler method) to complete the calculations.

Enter your BMR here: _____.

This is *without* exercise how many calories you need to consume to stay at your current weight. Use the lists on page 23 to judge the amount of calories you burn during exercise. Also remember that your BMR doesn't calculate how much lean body tissue you have . . . the more muscle you have, the higher your metabolism.

Beverages—Bad News, Good News

Before we get to how Molly modifies her diet, I want to address another important topic. I can't stress enough the importance of drinking enough water every day. You need water. Beyond keeping you alive, water helps in lots of other ways. Drinking the right amount of water helps satisfy you, which keeps you full, which leads to weight loss. It helps flush fat; and not only that, being properly hydrated makes your skin look purty!

Drinking water also reduces water retention. That seems kind of funny, doesn't it? Drinking more water makes your body retain less water? You would think it would do the opposite. Drinking enough water each day does make you have to pee more and that helps reduce the amount of water your body retains.

You may be thinking, "I know that, and I do drink water all the time." Well, if we are drinking water, then why do some studies suggest as many as 75 percent of Americans suffer from some degree of dehydration every day? In a recent survey participants were asked to describe their beverage consumption habits. Overall respondents averaged only 4.6 eight-ounce servings of water per day (most health and nutrition experts recommend at least eight servings of that size per day). Forty-four percent reported drinking only three servings or less per day. Yet paradoxically, the survey shows that Americans drink more water than any other type of beverage.

One of the most significant findings, however, was that while a typical American may consume eight servings of hydrating beverages each day, he or she also drinks five servings of dehydrating beverages in the same time frame. This results in a net gain of only three hydrating beverages per day. This is key because it suggests few Americans realize that hydrating and dehydrating beverages together can "cancel" each other out. Our bodies retain hydrating beverages and use the water in them in normal, healthy body processes. Bottled water, tap water, juice, milk, and carbonated soda without caffeine are all hydrating beverages. The most common dehydrating beverages are coffee, tea, carbonated soda with caffeine, beer, wine, and other alcoholic drinks. They are diuretics, meaning they promote fluid output, first in the form of increased urine production. Minor dehydration often results in fatigue, headache, facial muscle pain, and cramping.

When you begin to cut back your calorie consumption you may be tempted to use soda as a quick pick-me-up when you are slumping. A twelve-ounce can of Pepsi, for example, contains 150 calories. Keep in mind that you will not only pay the price in terms of excess calories, but that the diuretic effect will exact a toll on you as well. Sure, you'll experience that immediate sugar rush, but in the long run, that small benefit will be off-set by all the other effects and will put you in a cycle of needing another boost. So focus on drinking water in place of soda. If Americans reduced their soft drink consumption, our diabetes epidemic would be lessened considerably.

I also understand that eliminating soda is difficult for most people, so I do encourage diet soda in place of sugar-filled snacks. Diet sodas do have fewer calories. You will find me going to the convenience store a few times a week for a twenty-four-ounce diet soda with crushed ice (partly because my daughter likes the car and it puts her to sleep for naptime and my work time). So I do not recommend drinking six diet sodas a day, but one twenty-four-ounce diet soda certainly won't hurt as long as you make up for it in water consumption. (Just keep in mind—if you become pregnant, get rid of the artificial sweeteners!)

Losing weight comes down to burning more calories than you consume. I repeat: to lose weight you must burn more calories than you consume! From now on, I'm going to refer to this concept as creating a calorie deficit. Weight loss involves creating a calorie deficit.

Here's the deal. In order to lose one pound you have to have a calorie deficit of 3,500. The reason I don't guarantee you anything ridiculous like a ten-pound weight loss in a week is because that type of weight loss isn't healthy, it doesn't make you feel good, and, most important, it's not sustainable. While a few of us could manage that for a while, we'd soon hit the wall and experience diet fatigue, which leads to yo-yo weight gains and losses. And when you yo-yo, you lose fat and muscle, only to gain back fat. Muscle is gone. (And we need that muscle to increase metabolism!) Additionally, think of it this way: ten pounds in a week would translate into a 35,000-calorie deficit in seven days. That's 5,000 fewer calories consumed and burned each day than what you took in and burned the week before.

Please don't get me wrong. It's wonderful if you make the healthful choice and have the turkey sandwich or the veggie delight salad for lunch. I applaud you for that. But ultimately, you are going to have to alter your lifestyle, and *together* nutrition and exercise can do wonders for you. It will take time and dedication, and you will have to take responsibility for your own eating. But believe me: you'll be so much happier in two years when you don't even have to think about doing another "diet." This is a permanent plan! A bold but true statement . . . if you have not lost weight after the six-week jump start, 90 percent of the time it is because you are eating too much and the other 10 percent is due to eating too little.

My six-week nutrition plan is a great jump start to losing ten to fifteen pounds. That's right, six weeks, and not just one pound.

Instead of throwing a high-risk pass far down the field in a desperate attempt to score a quick touchdown, we're going to move down the field bit by bit. Why? Because we know what our long-term goal is, we've examined our own tendencies (strengths and weaknesses), and we know that based on past experience, and what researchers have learned about weight loss, slow and steady wins the race to shed and keep off excess weight. The numbers don't lie.

If Molly could give up her midmorning Pepsi, she'd cut 150 calories, and she'd be more than halfway to her 250-calorie-per-day deficit. She'd also be eliminating one of the diuretics from her diet, and her excuse about not wanting to drink as much water because of too many trips to the bathroom goes out the window!

Speaking of diuretics and beverages, for better or worse, Molly can't start her day without a cup of coffee. She usually has splurged for a medium latte with whole milk that checks in at 220 calories. In keeping her food diary, she discovered just how many calories she consumes each morning, and found that some of the more exotic blends and flavors of roasted beans, sugar, and sweetened dairy products could easily reach 1,000 calories. Opting out of her favorite sixteen ounces, she instead chose to have a slightly smaller latte (14 oz.) with skim milk, cutting the calorie content by more than half. That additional 120 calories pushes her total calorie cutting to 270.

Little adjustments can make a big difference down the line.

Mental Strategy

When you live your life in a constant state of *can't* (can't have this, can't have that) you set up a negative state of mind. That's not a good way for anyone to live their life. Negativity produces more negativity. After all, when we're cheering for our team, we're not chanting, "Don't fumble the ball! Don't fumble the ball!" You want to be positive and realistic. My motto has always been "It's not about making the best choices, it's about making the better choice."

What you will learn is that you can still eat fast food, still drink your favorite coffee, and still lose weight by making the *better* choice. Remember what I said about three weeks? Well, what happens a lot of the time is that when you develop the habit of making better choices, after three weeks of that, what had been your "better" choice now doesn't look as good as other alternatives out there and you make a *better* better choice! There are also ways to make up for your less-than-better choices. We aren't robots and we all crumble in the face of a delicious crumb cake every now and then. If you do, don't beat yourself up and create all kinds of negativity. Just take the next opportunity to make a better choice—instead of that Pepsi and Snickers bar (430 calories) have a glass of water and an apple (80 calories) and save yourself 350 calories. That 350-calorie savings should translate into 350 pats on the back as well.

I always had an extra five pounds that would come and go, especially when I was in college and had erratic eating patterns. Finally I wised up. I realized that I'm not a food martyr and that the occasional cheeseburger was something I had to have . . . and that I *liked* calorie-rich tuna salad. That's when I discovered the "don't tell yourself you can't" secret. I'd eat the cheeseburger or the tuna salad and then compensate for that at the next opportunity. Of course, I had to have the discipline to not skip on the compensating part. All of us have our weaknesses and our hormones sometimes give us cravings—whether we're the sweet or salty junk-food types. I recommend compensating by eating water-filled foods like soups and salads.

I love licorice. I could eat handfuls of the stuff all day. But I don't. I limit myself to consuming 150 calories of it. If I go out for a great dinner and top it off with a scrumptious dessert, I make more careful choices the next day or so to be sure I stay in control of my weight. The principle is simple. Instead of yo-yoing between one weight and another, using the bad day/good day system, your weight will remain steady.

For me, a good day starts with fruit for breakfast, yogurt for a snack, a chicken sandwich with a lot of veggie toppings and soup for lunch, almonds and a cheese stick for a snack, and a vegetable dinner. That veggie dinner is often a homemade baked potato with broccoli and cheese—2 percent cheese, of course! If you want to go out to dinner with friends and splurge a little, you can! Just get back on track the next day. You also need to teach yourself portion control and the push-away—when to push yourself or your plate away with that half-eaten cheeseburger and fries still in front of you. We'll talk more about portion control in a bit, but basically, I want you to feel good about yourself, your food intake, and your exercise routine. If you can do this six days a week, you will be well on your way to a healthy lifestyle.

A NOTE ON MEAL REPLACEMENT DRINKS AND BARS

I'm not convinced that most people need to go this route, but a simple and often effective way to cut calorie consumption and to be assured that you are getting all the right nutrients and macronutrients is to use meal replacement drinks. Some people don't like the taste of them and others don't like the expense, but one truth that can't be denied is that they work. More than thirty independent studies have shown that Slim-Fast in particular is an effective means of losing weight and, more important, keeping that weight off. The question is whether or not you want to spend the money and have the same thing to drink/eat at certain meals or snacks for that long.

Food for thought: these replacement bars and drinks are just that—a *replacement*. I find women adding them to their daily nutrition all the time. You can't add that number of calories to your diet; you have to use replacement drinks and bars in place of regular meals.

Product	Total Calories	Serving Size
Beverages	**Calories**	**Serving Size**
Slim-Fast Original	220	11 oz.
Slim-Fast Optima	190	11 oz.
Ensure Lite	200	8 oz.
Zone Perfect	260	8 oz.
Myoplex	120	11 oz.
Atkins	170	11 oz.
Met RX	170	11 oz.
Prolab Lean Mass Matrix	390	12–16 oz.
Bars*	**Calories**	**Fiber (Grams)**
Zone Bars	210	2
Balance Bars	200	1
Boulder Bar	200	5
Clif Bar	220	5
Luna Bar	180	2
PowerBar	230	3
Promax Bar	280	2

* I recommend choosing one that contains at least three grams of fiber.

This list isn't comprehensive, but it should give you some idea of what's out there. Life is all about making choices, and this can be another play you could put into your game plan.

Although you may cringe at the word "fiber," it is an important and essential nutrient. It also plays a huge part in weight loss. Why?

Fiber assists in filling you up, therefore discouraging overeating and helping in weight loss.

Getting enough daily fiber helps food move through the digestive system, and as an added benefit, it lowers cholesterol and prevents heart disease.

You need fiber in your diet for several other reasons. First, the body uses it to soften and add bulk to your stool—you will eliminate waste more easily. Second, high-fiber foods help you feel full longer while providing you with other nutrients. Complex carbohydrates are high in fiber and contain much-needed nutrients like B vitamins, vitamin C, vitamin K, iron, and folate. You should aim to eat twenty-five to thirty-five grams of fiber a day. Higher-fiber foods include whole-grain pastas, fruits with skin on, raw vegetables, whole-grain cereals, and whole-grain breads. Remember high grain = more fiber = more filling = less craving/hunger = less consumption.

A note on fiber. Slowly increase to that twenty-five to thirty-five grams a day—otherwise you will be bloated and uncomfortable! I learned this the hard way before my first cheerleading practice. I looked pregnant in my two-piece practice outfit after downing whole-wheat pasta with broccoli and fiber powder—yikes! Fiber powders are a good alternative for increasing fiber intake. But please read directions on label about how much to begin with.

How much fiber should you have in your diet?

- Kids—add five to your child's age (for example, a seven-year-old should get twelve grams of fiber)
- Adults (fifteen years and older)—twenty-five grams of fiber
- Pregnant women—twenty-five to thirty-five grams of fiber (thirty-five grams to relieve constipation that comes with pregnancy)

Here are some easy ways to incorporate more fiber into your family meals (and they don't just include broccoli and beans!).

Breakfast Ideas
- Incorporate fresh fruits.
- Make pancakes and waffles with whole-wheat mix. You can also add in berries for extra flavor.

- Eat whole-grain cereals. (Make sure whole grain is listed first in the ingredients.)
- Try whole-grain or whole-wheat toast and English muffins.
- Oatmeal is yummy and provides an average of 2.8 grams per serving.
- Mix your favorite cereal with a small amount of fiber-rich cereal.
- Mix almonds, apples, oranges, pears, bananas, and strawberries for a sweet crunch!

Lunch Ideas
- Leave the skins on your fruits and veggies for added fiber.
- Add a baked sweet potato to your normal salad or soup.
- Add almonds, black beans, or berries to your everyday salad.
- Make sandwiches with whole-grain breads. (Make sure whole grain is listed first in the ingredients.)
- Use whole-wheat tortillas to make your lunch. Roll cheese and turkey into tortillas, and cut into pieces for kids' finger foods. Wrap chicken, romaine lettuce, tomatoes, and your favorite dressing into your tortilla.

Dinner Ideas
- Make sure your plate is full of vegetables.
- Incorporate a baked potato with the skin to any meal. Make baked potato skins for the kids (quarter potato lengthwise and add low-fat shredded cheese).
- Use whole-grain pasta instead of regular pasta.
- Try the new flavored whole-grain rice side dishes or vegetables alongside chicken!
- Start with a green salad, or incorporate some greens into your meals.
- Try fresh fruit for dessert.

Begin with eating approximately ten grams of fiber consistently for three or four days then increase that amount by five grams every other day. If you start to feel uncomfortable bloating make sure you are not going overboard with the fiber and be sure you are drinking enough noncaffeinated fluids each day.

Drink at least eight eight-ounce glasses of noncaffeinated drinks daily to increase fiber's effect.

Get regular physical activity to stimulate the digestive tract and promote regular bowel movements.

It's Not Just How Much, It's What You Consume

So far in talking about nutrition, we've focused on how much you consume, how many calories you take in. In terms of weight loss, that's important but not the *only* thing to think about. You also need to consider your overall health and what you should consume to stay healthy. That means consuming calories from all food groups—grains, vegetables, fruits, healthy oils, meat or beans, and milk. And all those calories come from one of three types of calories: carbohydrates, fats, and protein. I list them in this order because it represents the highest to lowest amounts of calories you should consume from each group each day.

Carbohydrates: 40 to 60 percent

Fats: 20 to 30 percent

Protein: 10 to 20 percent

A typical meal is mostly made up of all three. For example, in a grilled cheese sandwich, the bread is carbs, the cheese is protein, and the olive oil and cheese are fats.

As you can see from my example above, my meal plans are not designed to get you to eat tofu and broccoli all the time. After all, it's about choosing better options and knowing that *best* options are still out there and available if you choose to go that way.

Far too many of us have protein at the top of our list. Most of us in this country consume twice this recommended amount of protein every day. Let's look at each of these three calorie sources individually.

CARBOHYDRATES

So much has been written about carbs in the past few years that most of us are confused about whether they are the devil's food or the angel's bread. So let's keep this simple: carbohydrates are essentially sugars. Your body needs them for fuel and they are the easiest form of fuel for the body to break down. You've all heard of the "sugar rush," right? Like the cookies our squad ate during halftime to give us a quick boost, sugary foods enable your body to metabolize (process) carbohydrates quickly to ensure an immediate rush of energy. Some carbohydrates are easier for your body to process and thus they produce a quick energy rush that eventually burns out. Those are called simple sugars. The sugar you spoon into your coffee, brown sugar, white bread, honey, candy—these are all simple sugars. They have a simple molecular structure that allows them to be processed quickly. You need some of these, but keep in mind their fast-starting, quickly burned-out nature. They don't last. That's why you slump after ingesting them. For that reason, experts in the medical/nutritional field have come to refer to them as "bad carbs." Simple carbs = bad carbs = hungry in thirty minutes.

Complex carbohydrates have a more complex molecular structure and it takes the body longer to metabolize them. You don't get the same nearly instantaneous rush from them that you get from the simple carbs. And because it takes longer for the body to metabolize them, you don't get the same rush-and-slump effect. The best part is, you don't get as hungry as quickly after consuming them. You can get complex carbohydrates from whole grains, vegetables, and legumes (beans). As my friend Stephanie Young, a registered dietitian, says, "You need complex carbohydrates because they add fiber, vitamins, and minerals to your diet. They also keep your blood sugar from experiencing the rapid highs and lows in simple carbohydrates. Complex carbohydrates are also usually lower in calories, saturated fat, and cholesterol. Plus, they make you feel fuller, longer!"

complex carbs = good carbs

So, the formula here is relatively simple. Limit the number of simple/bad carbs and increase the number of complex/good carbs in your diet. How do you do that? The Harvard University School of Public Health published this list of tips for adding good carbs to your diet:

1. Start the day with whole grains. Try a hot cereal, like old-fashioned oats, or a cold cereal that lists a whole grain first on the ingredient list.
2. Use whole-grain breads for lunch or snacks.
3. Bag the potatoes. Instead, try brown rice, bulgur, wheat berries, whole-wheat pasta, or another whole grain with your dinner. Those

are your best choices, but selecting a potato instead of buttered noodles is still a better choice.

4. Choose whole fruit instead of juice. An orange has two times as much fiber and half as much sugar as a twelve-ounce glass of orange juice.

5. Bring on the beans. Beans are an excellent source of slowly digested carbohydrates as well as a great source of protein.

You can check out the "What You Should Eat" portion of their website: www.hsph.harvard.edu/nutritionsource/what-should-you-eat. The Harvard School of Public Health's website is great and you don't have to be a Harvard graduate to understand it!

FATS

Just like carbohydrates, fats are a necessary part of nutrition. They do several things for our bodies: they help transport nutrients, they cushion our organs and joints, and they are an additional energy source. Just like carbohydrates, there are good fats and bad fats. The interesting thing about fats is that illness doesn't come from how *much* fat you consume, but from which *type* of fat you consume.

The "bad" fats—saturated and trans fats—increase the risk for certain diseases. The "good" fats—monounsaturated and polyunsaturated fats—lower disease risk. The key to a healthy diet is to substitute good fats for bad fats—and to avoid trans fats.

I don't want this to turn into a course on chemistry, but it is important to understand a few more facts about fat since for so long the low-fat diet was thought to be the great cure-all and weight reduction path. Remember my erratic eating patterns in college? I stocked my college dorm room with fat-free treats. I'd eat half a box of cookies because they were fat free. But they weren't calorie free! Fifteen pounds later I realized there is no way you can eat anything you want. You can consume plenty of calories in a fat-free food—almost 1,000 calories were in the half box of cookies I ate. Which didn't leave much room for me to fill up without going over my BMR. Almost everything we eat has some fat in it. Even carrots and lettuce have some fat content. That's how important they are to the body.

Good Fats

Unsaturated fats improve blood cholesterol levels, reduce inflammation, stabilize heart rhythms, and do other good things for your body. Foods from plants, such as vegetable oils, nuts, and seeds, are a good source of unsaturated fats. Unsaturated fats come in two types:

- Monounsaturated fats: canola, peanut, and olive oils; avocados; nuts such as almonds, hazelnuts, and pecans; and seeds such as pumpkin and sesame seeds.
- Polyunsaturated fats: sunflower, corn, soybean, and flaxseed oils, and also in foods such as walnuts, flaxseeds, and fish. (Omega-3 fats are an important type of polyunsaturated fat. The body can't make these, so they must come from food. An excellent way to get omega-3 fats is by eating fish two or three times a week.)

A lot of us stay away from things like avocados, nuts, and olive oil. We think they are too rich in fat and therefore bad for us. That's not the case. We need their mono- and polyunsaturated fats. Try these to add good fats to your eating:

- Instead of cream cheese on your bagel, try almond or peanut butter.
- Try pumpkin seeds, sunflower seeds, or almonds on your salad instead of croutons. Less than what would fill the cup of your hand is a good portion.
- Sauté your favorite vegetables in olive oil instead of butter.

Bad Fats

Our bodies produce all the saturated fat we need. That's why we should avoid eating foods that contain them. Our saturated fats come mainly from meat, seafood, and whole-milk dairy products (cheese, milk, and ice cream). A few plant foods are also high in saturated fats, including coconut and coconut oil, palm oil, and palm kernel oil. Look for these oils in ingredients lists and limit your intake of foods that contain them.

Very Bad Fats

Food manufacturers want their products to stay fresh on the shelves longer. For that reason, they began using trans-fatty acids (trans fats) in their recipes. By heating vegetable oil in the presence of hydrogen gas, a process called hydrogenation, they make the oil more stable so it won't spoil as quickly. Because they are more stable, hydrogenated fats can be used again and again, so fast-food companies use them to fry their foods.

You Really Can Eat What You Want—in Moderation

Portion control is probably the most important thing when looking at your current eating habits. You may know pizza is not the best meal solution, but you can eat it in moderation. Just be sure that you eat plenty of fruits and vegetables throughout the rest of the day. Society as a whole, and restaurants in particular, skew our sense of correct portions. I will teach you an easy method for judging portion sizes (using your hand) later on.

Stay away from diet pills and anything else that promises quick results—they're a gimmick. You *have* to eat well and exercise to lose weight and to improve health. That's all I have to say about diet pills (somehow they gross more money than any fitness DVD).

Any time you see the words "hydrogenated" or "partially hydrogenated" on a food label, it means that there are trans fats in that food product. The average American eats about six grams of trans fats a day. Ideally that should be under two grams a day, or zero if possible. A new labeling law that requires food companies to list trans fats on the label should help you keep track of and avoid the foods that have trans fats in them. Most of the trans fats we eat come from commercially prepared baked goods, margarines, snack foods, and processed foods, along with french fries and other fried foods prepared in restaurants and fast-food franchises. The quick rule of thumb is that the more processed a food is, the better off you are avoiding it. But if snack crackers are your thing, I am not going to tell you to eliminate them; I just want you to be aware of what you are taking in.

1. To avoid bad fats, the Harvard School of Public Health suggests that you use liquid plant oils for cooking and baking. Olive, canola, and other plant-based oils are rich in heart-healthy unsaturated fats. Try dressing up a salad or spring vegetables with a delicious olive oil–based vinaigrette.
2. Ditch the trans fats. In the supermarket, read the labels to find foods that are free of trans fats. In restaurants, steer clear of fried foods, biscuits, and other baked goods, unless you know that the restaurant has eliminated trans fats. Read more about how to spot trans fats—and how to avoid them.
3. Switch from butter to soft tub margarine. Choose a product that has zero grams of trans fats, and scan the ingredient list to make sure it does not contain partially hydrogenated oils.
4. Eat at least one good source of omega-3 fats each day. Fatty fish like salmon, walnuts, and canola oil all provide omega-3 fatty acids.
5. Go lean on meat and milk. Beef, pork, lamb, and dairy products are high in saturated fat. Choose low-fat milk, and savor full-fat cheeses in small amounts; also, choose lean cuts of meat.

PROTEIN

As with the other two main sources of calories, protein actually has both good and bad components. Protein itself is a good and necessary part of our diet. It plays an important role in transporting oxygen to our cells, among other things, and we have to take in protein every day because unlike fats and carbs, our body doesn't store protein. The trouble with protein for most of us is that, first, we eat too much of it, and second, protein doesn't exist in a pure state. By that I mean that when you eat, for example, a six-ounce chunk of beef like a porterhouse steak, you're also getting forty-four grams of fat. That's a lot of fat! So even if you manage to eat just the right amount of protein, you might be getting too much of other bad things. So what's a girl to do? You could become a vegetarian and avoid all meat and dairy products entirely. That would be helpful, but vegetarianism can make proper protein consumption a little tricky. There are complete proteins, which contain all of the necessary amino acids (the building blocks of protein), and incomplete proteins, which lack some of those essential building blocks. Meat and fish are complete proteins. The proteins found in things like fruits, vegetables, grains, and nuts are incomplete. There are some twenty amino acids that you need, and you have to get about half of them from your food; your body doesn't make them. So if you aren't eating complete proteins, you need to vary your diet (a good idea in any case) to get enough of those particular amino acids into your system.

The best sources of protein (because what they contain is also healthier) are poultry and fish. Red meat is not the best for you, but you may need some of it for the reasons I cited above. For most people, a few ounces of red meat two or three times a week is enough to give them the "complete" protein package they need.

Keep in mind that proteins are also calorie rich. That six-ounce steak I mentioned? It can contain as much as half of your daily calorie intake re-

---

MEET A MEMBER OF THE FAMILY

Bethany has been a St. Louis Rams Cheerleader for three years. Here are some tips she shares about nutrition:

"I generally eat what I want but in moderation. I try to make sure that I don't get stuck eating the same types of meals all the time. If I have chicken one night, then I'll do fish the next or a pasta dish. I eat frozen vegetables, green salads, and lots of fruit. I also make sure to get fiber by changing my breakfast routine. I usually go back and forth between cereal and eggs/toast. I also try to eat dinner as early as possible—usually, no later than 7:30 p.m. if my schedule permits. Also, I keep fruit as a snack during the day. I usually start feeling hungry by 3:30 p.m., so I'll have a nice serving of fruit to get me through the remainder of the afternoon. And of course, lots of water. As much water as I can stand (sometimes that's not much). I stay away from sodas and generally drink juice and water. Don't get me wrong. I do enjoy the good stuff like burgers, fries, and ice cream, but always in moderation. That's the key."

quirement. And one piece of fried chicken from your favorite spot? Enough protein to meet your daily requirement!

Also keep in mind that there are many foods high in protein that are not chicken, beef, fish, or poultry. Nuts, legumes, dairy, eggs, and grains contain protein. As with all other food groups, you get more than just protein when you consume them.

Food Packaging Labels

If you are going to be keeping track of what you eat and what nutrients it contains and in what amounts, you're going to be doing a lot of reading of packages and labels. The nutrition labels are fairly straightforward, but food manufacturers sometimes use buzz words that can be confusing and our own lack of understanding adds to that. Here's a list of those words and an explanation of what they mean:

- Free: The product contains an insignificant amount of a particular nutrient. Our confusion comes in when we mistake fat free with calorie free. For example, pretzels are fat free but they aren't calorie free.
- Reduced: The product contains 25 percent less of a nutrient or total calories than the "regular" product. Again, this doesn't mean fewer calories.
- Light: The product contains 33 percent fewer calories *or* 50 percent of the fat content of the original product. While this is a good thing, eating more of a light product negates the weight loss or health benefits.
- Lean: The meat product contains less than ten grams of fat and 4.5 grams or less of saturated fat.
- Good source: One serving of that food contains 10 percent to 19 percent of that particular nutrient.
- Whole grain: The word "whole" must come before "grain." Nine-grain or seven-grain doesn't mean whole. You want whole grain.

Reviewing the Highlights

- Know your numbers: your BMI, your BMR, and your weight.
- Keep track of what you consume in a food diary.
- To lose weight, burn more calories and take in fewer calories.
- A calorie is a calorie whether it comes from a cheeseburger or whole-wheat pasta.
- Eat high-volume foods to stay fuller and satisfied longer.
- Learn portion control—the palm method will be explained in chapter 4.
- You don't always have to eat the best choices to lose weight. A few "better" choices will do!
- It is essential to eat a variety of foods within each group: grains, fruits, vegetables, protein, dairy, and fats.

Remember, it's all about the number of calories you consume! Let's decide to go for the *best* choice over the next six weeks during your jump-start phase. Choose fruit instead of a cookie and be on your way to losing weight . . . isn't that why you bought the book?

EATING ON THE RUN

Now it's time to put all this useful information to work for us. Most of us eat more than our BMR requirement, or needed calories, for the day. Whatever your reason for taking in more calories than your BMR, my goal for you is to get in the ballpark of your BMR during your first twenty-four hours of eating while following my guidelines. Although you probably will not lose a pound or gain a pound in that first twenty-four-hour period, if you consume approximately the number of calories equal to your BMR for seven days straight and add exercise you will lose weight. The Nutrition Jump Start will get you in that ballpark. Add in the exercise plan and there you go!

Nutrition Jump Start + six-week zone interval training = weight loss

Think about it for a minute. Go back to chapter 3 and record the BMR figure you calculated for yourself here: _____.

Lindsay's Shortcut Method for Eating Right

Before I became a St. Louis Rams Cheerleader, I worked with the squad as a kickboxing instructor. Keep this in mind: the women I trained (and who I later cheered with) were a lot like you. There were some exceptions, but most of the women on the squad held down other jobs and didn't spend all their time working out in a gym. Many of them had children in addition to their careers. They all wanted to be fit, but they also wanted to have fun and full lives apart from being cheerleaders. That meant that they were, like you, looking for easy ways to incorporate good eating practices and exercise into their busy lives.

For those of you who find calorie counting too time-consuming, I am going to give you the specifics for my shortcut portion control system. Remember, there are two parts to good nutrition: what you eat and how much of it you eat. Most of us underestimate the size of the servings (portions) we consume. That's one reason why I want you to keep a food journal and track your calories. Some of you may not have the time to do both these things. *Do not give up the food journal.* I'd rather have you track what you eat and not calculate the specific calorie content of the foods you consume than the other way around.

I'm also not going to give you elaborate meal plans. What I will provide you with is something you can easily incorporate into your life today without making too many adjustments, preparing new grocery lists, etc. My plan makes eating the right amount and the right foods fast and easy.

As a part of my shortcut, you will measure the amount you eat using the palm method. This will give you an approximate "correct" portion of each item from the food groups listed below.

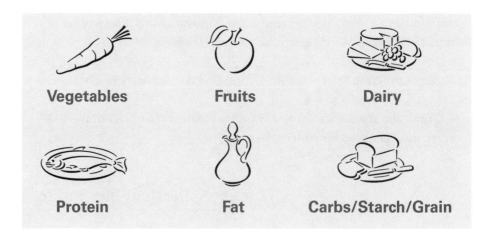

Vegetables   **Fruits**   **Dairy**

Protein   **Fat**   **Carbs/Starch/Grain**

As you can see, I've used icons to represent each group. On page 70 you'll find an example of the food journal I've provided at the back of the book, where you will see these icons in the daily tracking sheets. Use these pages provided in the book for your first week of the Cheerleader Fitness Plan. This is to get you started. Please visit my website to print out the sheets for the next five weeks of the plan at www.momsintofitness.com. If you want to continue using the food journal after you've completed the Cheerleader Fitness Plan, you can download more blank pages from my website.

The Food Journal

I said at the very beginning of this book that my Ultimate Six-Week Fitness Plan is a way for you to make a lifestyle change. Instead of just temporarily changing your behavior and then abandoning what you learned and what you did, my plan will help you to make the more exercise- and nutrition-conscious state of mind and being you have developed into your "new normal." I'm not the first person to use that term, and a lot of self-help and personal improvement books and their authors talk about this concept. This is a change that can last a lifetime.

Basically, what I'm hoping is that you will experience the kinds of changes in your body that you wanted. As a result, you'll want to stick with this "new" you and continue to work out and eat in a way that allows you to maintain the weight you targeted for yourself. I also understand that there will be times when you won't be able to work out, and there will be times when you will indulge some of your cravings. Please continue to use my program to get back on track quickly and easily when you need it most.

One of the keys to success is the food journal. Here is the blank journal that you will use to track your daily consumption.

· Food Journal ·

Breakfast: _____
_____
_____

Time:_____

Snack: _____
_____

Time:_____

Lunch: _____
_____
_____

Time:_____

Snack: _____
_____

Time:_____

Dinner: _____
_____
_____

Time:_____

Check off the icons to track the number of units of each food group you're consuming. And remember to record your measurements weekly—the largest circumference of your arm, chest, hips, thigh, one inch above belly button, and one inch below belly button—and measure the same exact spot each week.

Become a Servant of the Serving: The Palm Method

When do you stop eating? If the answer is that you are a lifetime member of the Clean Plate Club, you might get brownie points from your mom, but you could also develop an unhealthy set of love handles. I'm not saying that you should waste food, but you should take a look at how much it is you are putting on your plate to polish off. Don't think that the size of the portions you get in restaurants is in any way, shape, or form healthy for you. Those oohs and aahs you let out when your server brings your plate to the table should be ughs and oh nos! The typical American serving size at home and when we dine out overserves us by three to four times. Put another way, that combo platter at your favorite local Mexican restaurant could contain as many calories as you need to take in for a full day—or more.

Helpful hint: *always* pack half your meal at a restaurant to take home or split an entrée with a meal partner.

How do you know what a serving or correction portion is? I teach my clients the palm method. Here's how you do it.

For carbohydrates one serving is one cupped palmful. Take your open hand and turn it over so that the palm is facing up. Cup your hand slightly. Next, pour in enough rice, pasta, or sliced potato to fill that curved palm. That's your serving. For most people, a palmful is about 200 calories.

Use a flat palm for proteins (fish, chicken, red meat, nuts, dairy, and legumes): your palm flat (palm only, no fingers), not cupped, is the same size as a correct serving of a protein food. A palm-size slice of chicken or red meat or fish will be anywhere from 150 to 400 calories. Make sure you read the label or go online for a calorie counter listing of that particular item.

**Carbohydrates:
Fill that curved palm.**

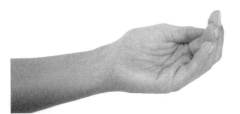

**Protein:
The size of a flat palm.**

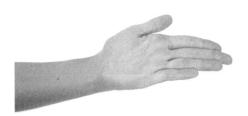

For fats, you should consume one to two "thumbs." This means that when you use oils in your cooking, pour an amount that will spread out to an area about the size of one or two of your thumbs. That one serving will equal about 200 calories.

**Fats:
One to two
thumbs.**

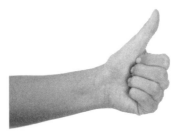

One serving of fruits and vegetables is equal to about the size of your fist. A fist of fruits or vegetables contains approximately 20 to 80 calories. Those apples the size of a softball are likely two fists. (If you were to spread some peanut butter—chiefly a fat—on that apple, you'd be consuming two fists and a thumb.)

**Fruits and Vegetables:
A fist. "A fist of fruits
or vegetables."**

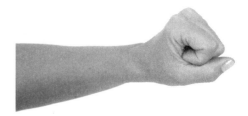

The size of the apple or other vegetable does matter in this sense. The reason why I say that you should eat more fruits and vegetables is that they are high-volume foods. They make you feel fuller sooner. You'll feel fuller from eating a smaller serving of fresh fruit and vegetables than you will from eating similar size portions of other foods.

Finally, for dairy products, a serving of liquid is equal to a fist-size portion and a thumb-size portion of solids like cheese. Both are equal to approximately 100 calories.

An Ideal Day of Eating

For the first three weeks of the Nutrition Jump Start, you should consume three small meals a day and one to two snacks. Your BMR is likely to fall within a range of calories—from 1,100 to 1,600. If you are a small- to medium-size woman, you are most likely to have a BMR that falls somewhere within this range. If you are a large-framed woman, you will need to consume more, so I recommend that you have one additional starch (one hand-cupping portion) and one additional portion of protein. You should never lower your calorie consumption below 1,000!

YOUR DAILY CONSUMPTION FROM EACH GROUP

1. Five servings of vegetables.
2. Three servings of fruit.
3. Two servings of dairy.
4. Two to three servings of protein.
5. One to two servings of fats.
6. Three servings of carbohydrates (starches and grains).

APPROXIMATE CALORIE CONSUMPTION
FROM EACH GROUP

Vegetables: Those five servings will account for 150 to 200 calories. One-half cup of cooked veggies or 1 cup of raw veggies is equal to approximately 30 calories. That's a lot of food in terms of weight, but not a lot in terms of calories. That's why I recommend you eat more vegetables. They add a lot of bulk in your stomach so you feel fuller, but they don't add a high calorie count.

Fruits: Your three servings of fruit will have you consuming 180 to 300 calories. As you can see, that's comparatively a lot more calories than vegetables. You can eat two more servings of vegetables and still end up 100 calories or so short of the number of calories you'd consume from eating fruit. Why? Generally, fruits have a higher sugar content than vegetables. Those sugars are good sources of instant energy and therefore more calorie rich. A palmful of grapes contains anywhere from 60 to 100 calories.

Dairy: Two servings from this group will give you about 200 calories, likely from milk (try 2 percent or skim because they are lower in fat and have more nutrients), cheese, or yogurt. An eight-ounce glass of milk contains about 100 calories, as does a thumb-size piece of cheese, a small yogurt cup, a small pudding cup, or a cup of soy milk. It's always good to be taking a multivitamin. Most women do not consume the 1,000–1,200 milligrams of calcium needed in a day. If you're consuming two dairy servings with this plan you are getting anywhere from 600 to 800 milligrams of calcium.

Protein: Your two to three servings of protein will provide you with between 300 and 600 calories. Ideally, you will get some protein from other sources besides red meat. If you do choose red meat, opt for leaner cuts. Generally, any "loin" cut of meat is leaner than other cuts. Loin contains approximately 200 calories in a three-ounce portion. Less-lean cuts contain about 300 calories in a three-ounce portion. Here are some other calorie equivalents for other protein sources. Each of these is equal to approximately 150 calories: one cup of beans, three-quarters cup of cottage cheese, one palmful of nuts, three-quarters cup of 2 percent shredded cheese, two tablespoons of peanut butter, fifteen small shrimp, three medium- or two large-size eggs, and a palm-size piece of chicken, pork, or fish.

Fats: The smallest amount of calories of any group should come from fats. The 100 calories you should consume can come from lots of sources, but remember what I said early on about good, bad, and very bad fats. Many types of nuts are a source of good protein, but mostly when they are eaten raw or dry roasted. One tablespoon of extra-virgin olive oil equals approximately 100 calories, as does half an avocado, one tablespoon of mayonnaise, one tablespoon of olive oil and vinegar salad dressing, and eight olives.

Carbohydrates (Grains and Starches): I mentioned earlier the importance of eating whole grains. Don't be deceived by "seven-grain" or "nine-grain" on the label. They are often not whole grains, so look for the word "whole" in the ingredients list when deciding what to consume to get your 300-calorie total for this group. One starch is equivalent to 100 calories and that is the caloric equivalent of one-half cup of pasta, potatoes, or rice, or two slices of whole-wheat bread, half of a whole-wheat pita, or a small baked white potato.

Some Things to Note

My suggested intake above doesn't list any calorie-rich beverages like regular soda, fruit juice, or alcohol. It also doesn't include potato chips, cookies, and alcoholic beverages or other "empty" calorie foods I mentioned earlier. Just because they aren't listed doesn't mean they are "forbidden." I just ask you to cut back and to keep track of them in your food journal. Some of us have that salty/oily thing going on and others of us have the sweet tooth happening. In general, you should limit your consumption of simple sugars and/or salty-oilies to less than 150 calories a day. If you can't quit on most days, at least commit to cutting back.

One of the things you have to learn is to feel full with your stomach and not with your eyes. If I were to put a small serving of your favorite fast-food french fries in front of you I bet you would eat less than if I had put a large-size portion in front of you. You would feel full, but your eyes would tell you there's more there. The Clean Plate Club was a good idea when you were a kid and you were being encouraged to eat all your veggies, but that habit may have had a bad long-term effect on you. I believe in clean plates, but as I mention above, your plate should start with high-bulk vegetables covering half of it.

The Vegetarian

Vegetarians often struggle to include enough protein in their diet; however, with careful planning a vegetarian diet can be healthy and safe. The first thing for you to do is to inform your health-care provider of your dietary habits. You may want to visit with a registered dietitian if you would like personalized meal planning or have specific concerns. Good protein sources for vegetarians include legumes, nuts, and seeds. The most important thing is to focus on variety and adequate calories in your diet. Vegetarians can also lack iron, calcium, and vitamin B_{12}. Please make sure to research with a professional ways to get nutrients you may lack.

Snacking

I recommend that you incorporate two snacks into your daily routine. Here's a list of possible snacks and their Lindsay unit equivalents:

4 cups light popcorn (season with cheese sprinkles for cheddar popcorn) = 1 starch

1 cup low-fat pudding (try strawberries dipped in chocolate pudding) = 1 dairy, 1 fruit

1 cup low-fat yogurt with sprinkles of crunchy cereal = 1 dairy, ½ starch

1 medium sweet potato = 1 vegetable

1 cup applesauce = 1 fruit

1 medium apple with one tablespoon peanut butter = 1 fruit, ½ protein, ½ fat

12 cocktail shrimp = 1 protein

1 medium baked potato with low-fat sour cream = 1 starch, 1 dairy

Handful almonds = 1 protein, 1 fat

12 whole-grain crackers with low-fat cheese = 1 starch, 1 dairy

2 pieces whole-grain bread with one tablespoon peanut butter = 1 starch, ½ protein, ½ fat

1 English muffin with one tablespoon peanut butter = 1 starch, ½ protein, ½ fat

Small salad with oil-based dressing = 1 vegetable, 1 fat

Veggies and hummus = 2 vegetable, ½ protein

Banana slices with one tablespoon peanut butter = 1 fruit, ½ protein, ½ fat

As I mentioned before, the first three weeks of any lifestyle change are always the hardest. I hope you see that I've designed a plan that will minimize the amount of adjustments you will have. When you see the results, I promise you, you will truly be motivated to continue on to the next three weeks. But please don't get discouraged if you don't see the results you want. As I've pointed out before, it's important to have realistic expectations. A pound or so at the beginning is about what you can expect in Phase 1. There are many variables that will contribute to your success. Concentrate on controlling the variables you can—what and how much you eat, and how much effort you put into your exercise days.

Choosing Wisely

Making a lifestyle change like the one you've committed to in buying this book and following my plan is all about making better choices. When it comes to nutrition, we all know that eating fast food is not the *best* option. But you can find better options when you go to your favorite fast-food place. I am not going to ask you to eliminate fast food or your favorite restaurant. We live in a fast-paced world and it's not always possible to cook a healthy meal at home (although I'd like you to try!). You could simply choose a salad with light dressing or a grilled chicken sandwich with small fries or a kid's meal. Ordering pizza for dinner? Sure, but stay away from pepperoni, sausage, and cheese-filled crust, and get one that is loaded with veggies and has a whole-wheat crust instead of one made from white flour. Oh, and you don't need that extra cheesy bread.

Here's a quick list of some typical fast-food offerings and their serving equivalents:

1. Salad with grilled chicken and oil dressing = 2 vegetable, 1 fat, 1 protein
2. Plain baked potato and side salad = 1 starch, 1 vegetable
3. Soups = 1 starch, 1 fat, 1 dairy (cream based), or 1 vegetable (broth based)
4. Grilled chicken sandwich (no mayo) and side salad = 1 starch, 1 protein, 1 vegetable, 1 fat
5. Try to steer clear of the hamburgers and french fries . . . but if you're going to do it, order a kid's meal = 2 starch, 1 protein, 2 fat
6. Turkey submarine sandwich (six inches) on whole-wheat bread = 1–2 starch, 1 protein, 1 dairy, 1 fat
7. Vegetable pizza (size small, or 2 slices of medium pizza) = 1 vegetable, 2 starch, 2 dairy, 1 protein, 1 fat
8. Bean burrito = 1 starch, 1 protein, 1 dairy, 1 fat
9. One milk shake = 3 starch, 2 dairy, 2 fat
10. One fried chicken breast, green beans, mashed potatoes = 2 protein, 3 fat, 2 starch, 1 vegetable

Dining Out

Fast food isn't the only form of dining out—who doesn't like going to a favorite restaurant for a relaxing meal? I want you to eat a variety of food groups, and sometimes to get an additional kind of variety, it helps to go somewhere that serves a particular cuisine. Most non-American cuisines are less protein/meat based, so you shouldn't have any trouble with getting the proper food groups in the proper proportions. Here's a list of cuisines and better options and other considerations for you when you dine out. I have also listed their serving equivalents to help you track how much to consume.

MEXICAN

Tips

1. Try to skip the chips.
2. Use salsa for extra flavor and steer clear of sour cream and cheese.

Treats and Tracking

- Two chicken fajitas with everything but sour cream and melted cheese = 2 protein, 2 starch, 1 dairy, 1 vegetable, 1 fat
- Two chicken tacos = 1 protein, 1 dairy, 2 starch, 1 vegetable, 1 fat
- Rice and beans (in moderation) = 2 starch, ½ protein
- Bean tostada = 1 starch, ½ protein, 1 dairy, ½ vegetable
- Beef taco = 1 starch, 1 protein, 1 dairy, 1 fat

ITALIAN

Tips

1. If you are going to have Italian bread, save it for your meal. Try not to snack on bread before you get your entrée.

Treats and Tracking

- Small vegetable pizza made with half of the cheese = 2–3 starch, 2 dairy, 2 vegetable, 1 fat, 1 protein
- One cup pasta with marinara or tomato sauce (whole-wheat pasta if possible) = 2 starch, 1 vegetable
- Salad and lunch-size beef spaghetti = 1 vegetable, 2 starch, 1 protein, 1 fat
- Broiled chicken and veggies = 1 protein, 2 vegetables, 1 fat
- Shrimp primavera (take half home) = 1 protein, 2 starch, 2 vegetable

ASIAN

Tips

1. Choose anything poached or steamed or lightly stir-fried.
2. Take advantage of the seafood items.
3. Side items can make a meal.

- Steamed vegetables = 2–3 vegetables
- Steamed rice or brown rice = 2 starch
- Half orders of broiled chicken (not fried . . . make sure to ask) = 1 protein
- Four steamed spring rolls = 1 starch, 1 vegetable

FRENCH

Tips

1. Choose wine-based sauces instead of cream-based sauces.
2. Choose nonfried appetizers, lightly sautéed.

Treats and Tracking

- Steamed mussels = 1 protein
- French onion soup with cheese = 2 dairy, 2 fat, 1–2 starch

GREEK

Tips

1. Yogurt-based sauces are better than cream-based sauces.

Treats and Tracking

- Chicken pita sandwich = 2 starch, 1 protein, 1 vegetable, 1 fat
- Shish kabob = 1–2 protein, 1–2 vegetable
- Three tablespoons couscous and veggies = 1 starch, ½ protein, 1 vegetable
- Dolma = 1 protein, 1 fat, 1 vegetable

STEAKHOUSE

Tips

1. Look for the word "loin" for leaner steaks.
2. Go for the soup and salad combo or a salad and a vegetable side.

Treats and Tracking

- Side salad, no cheese, with dressing on the side = 1 vegetable, 1 fat
- Baked potato and steamed vegetables = 1 starch, 2 vegetable
- Palm-size serving of lean steak with steamed vegetables = 1 protein, 1 vegetable, 1 fat
- Plain baked chicken or seafood = 1 protein, 1 fat
- Peel-and-eat shrimp = 1 protein (cocktail sauce: add 1 starch)

BREAKFAST

Tips

1. One small box of cereal with skim milk will give you lots of nutrients at a low calorie cost.
2. Have your eggs made with egg whites or Egg Beaters.

Treats and Tracking

- Omelet made with two eggs, veggies, and a small amount of cheese = 1 protein, 1 vegetable, 1 dairy, 1 fat
- Two pieces toast or English muffin = 1 starch
- Waffle topped with fruit = 2 starch, 1 fruit
- Cereal with skim milk = 1 starch, 1 dairy
- Cottage cheese and fruit = 1 protein, 1 fruit
- Two pancakes and turkey bacon = 1½ starch, 1½ dairy, ½ protein, 1 fat

DINING OUT RULES

1. Choose clear broth soups like chicken noodle or minestrone to fill you up.
2. Start with a small side salad (dressing on the side).
3. Package half of your plate "to go."
4. A meal can be made up of side items such as: side salad, baked potato, vegetables, beans, pilafs, shrimp cocktail, soup, etc.
5. When ordering meat, fish, or poultry, make sure it's steamed, baked, grilled, broiled, roasted, or poached—*not fried*.
6. Avoid menu items with the words "creamy," "cheesy," "breaded," or "batter-dipped" in them.
7. Avoid casseroles and gravy (or heavy sauce).
8. Have tea or coffee for dessert.
9. No buffets.
10. *Forget* jumbo, large, supersize, etc.

With this guide in mind, you can choose sensibly when you hear, "May I take your order, please?" I think you get the idea by now.

Your Own Fast Food at Home

An easy fast-food option that doesn't require you to go out is to have a lean frozen meal and a side salad or veggie. There are a number of good lean/low-calorie options in your local grocery store. I know that at mine, I'm seeing more and more organic options in the frozen food aisle as well. Anything you can do to cut down on the number of preservatives and other chemicals is always a good thing to do.

One of the best options for fast food on days when you're too busy to cook is to prepare your meals on Sundays and have them prepackaged and ready to go. You can do this with wraps, sandwiches, and soups most easily, but you can convert any meal into homemade fast food pretty easily.

I don't want to send you to the grocery store with a list full of meal plans, so find a recipe or two from the ones I've collected and try the one that most tempts you!

All the recipes in this chapter and elsewhere in the book are based on my plate method or nutrition plan, which means they are full of veggies and lean meats. *Plus* they can all be made in ten to thirty minutes!

✤ A Different Kind of "Fast Food"...

1. "Light" or "low-fat" TV dinner served with a side of vegetables
2. Homemade grilled cheese sandwich and a cup of soup
3. Express bagged salad
4. Crackers, turkey, and cheese
5. Fresh soup from the grocery store

✤ Chicken in 10!

INGREDIENTS

    1 rotisserie chicken from the local grocery store
    1 package frozen green beans
    1 package whole-grain rice
    1 tablespoon olive oil
    Pinch of garlic salt

Remove skin from chicken. Place green beans in ⅓ cup water in a micro-wave-safe bowl or steamer. Use a microwave-safe lid on the bowl or steamer and steam on high for 6 minutes. Cook whole-grain rice on the stove according to package directions. Slice the rotisserie chicken into 4-ounce portions (about the size of your palm). Drain green beans and toss in olive oil, top with a pinch of garlic salt. (Remember, vegetables should take up half of your plate!)

Makes four servings at approximately 350 calories per serving.

❖ Men Eat Salad . . . with Wing Sauce

INGREDIENTS

  2 chicken breasts (no skin)
  Seasoned coating mix for chicken (my husband prefers Shake 'N Bake
    Extra Crispy)
  1 bag of your favorite salad mix
  1 green pepper
  ½ cup of your favorite cheese (I use reduced fat feta cheese)
  4 tablespoons wing sauce
  Tortilla chips (optional)

Preheat oven to 400 degrees. Prepare the chicken according to the seasoned coating mix directions. Prepare two plates with salad, cut-up green pepper, and cheese. Cut the chicken into strips and coat with wing sauce. Serve chicken over the salad and crumble tortilla chips on top.

Makes two servings at approximately 300 calories per serving without chips.

❖ Zucchini Stix

INGREDIENTS

  4–5 tablespoons dry bread crumbs (seasoned or unseasoned)
  2 tablespoons Parmesan cheese
  1 egg white
  1 teaspoon milk
  2 small zucchini, cut lengthwise into quarters
  ½ cup your favorite spaghetti sauce

Combine bread crumbs and Parmesan cheese. Combine egg white and milk in another dish. Dip each zucchini stick into both mixtures and place on baking sheet. Coat with cooking spray and bake for 15 minutes at 400 degrees. Serve with sauce.

Makes eight stix at approximately 30 calories each.

❖ Secret Pizza

1 16-ounce packaged pizza crust
1½ cups low-fat mozzarella cheese
4 cups pureed vegetables
1 jar pizza sauce

Simply blend any of your favorite—and your family's least favorite—veggies into the pizza sauce and cover with a concealing layer of cheese. About 4 cups of veggie to one cookie sheet. Spinach works very well in this recipe.

Makes eight slices at approximately 200 calories per slice.

❖ Mexican Soup in 15 Minutes

INGREDIENTS

1 pound lean (5/95) ground beef
1 package ranch dressing mix
1 package reduced-sodium taco seasoning mix
2 cups water (you can vary this for thinner or thicker soup)
1 can diced tomatoes and green chilies (15 oz.)
1 can stewed tomatoes (16 oz.)
1 can whole-kernel white corn (16 oz.)
1 can chili beans, rinsed and drained (15 oz.)

In a browning pan or skillet, heat the lean ground beef until cooked thoroughly. Once the beef cooking is under way, begin heating a pot (medium size) of water on medium-high heat. Add diced tomatoes, stewed tomatoes, corn, and beans. Once the beef is fully cooked, drain excess liquid, then add ranch and taco mixes to the beef. Add beef mix to the soup pot and simmer to heat through. Enjoy!

Makes four servings at approximately 300 calories per serving.

❖ Chicken Salad

INGREDIENTS

    10 boneless, skinless, frozen chicken breast tenderloins
    ⅓ cup light sour cream
    ⅔ cup light mayonnaise
    ½ cup chopped celery (or to taste)
    ⅓ cup chopped green onion (or to taste)
    Grapes (optional)
    Whole-wheat pitas or wraps (optional)

Bake the chicken at 350 degrees for 20–25 minutes, remove from oven, and let the chicken cool before breaking it into small pieces. In a large mixing bowl, combine chicken, light sour cream, light mayo, chopped celery, chopped green onion, and grapes (optional). Chill and serve with mini whole-wheat pitas or whole-wheat wraps.

Without the pita wrap this makes ten servings at approximately 150 calories each.

❖ Meatless Chili—for Vegetarians and Nonvegetarians

INGREDIENTS

    1 medium onion, chopped
    4 cloves garlic, minced
    1 tablespoon olive oil
    ½ cup shredded carrots
    1 can stewed tomatoes
    1 can diced tomatoes
    2 cans black beans, rinsed and drained
    ½–1 package chili seasoning mix
    1 tablespoon chopped parsley

Sauté onions and garlic in oil in a pan large enough for remaining ingredients. Add carrots, tomatoes, beans, seasoning mix, and parsley. Cook on medium heat for 10–15 minutes.

Makes three servings at approximately 250 calories per serving.

✣ Pasta Fazool

INGREDIENTS
   1 pound lean (5/95) ground beef
   1 cup diced onion
   1 cup sliced celery
   1 cup sliced carrots
   2 cloves minced garlic
   1 can tomatoes (15 oz.)
   1 can tomato sauce (15 oz.)
   1 can red kidney beans, undrained (15 oz.)
   2 cups water
   5 teaspoons beef bouillon
   1 tablespoon dried parsley flakes
   1 teaspoon salt
   ½ teaspoon oregano
   ½ teaspoon sweet basil
   ¼ teaspoon black pepper
   ½ cup small macaroni

Brown beef in large skillet and drain. Add all ingredients except macaroni, bring to a boil. Lower heat, cover, and simmer 20 minutes. Add macaroni and return to boil. Simmer until vegetables are done (10 minutes). If your kids don't like it, freeze it in small containers for a quick lunch.

Makes six servings at approximately 220 calories per serving.

❖ Mexican Chicken Soup

INGREDIENTS

    4 cups chicken broth
    1 cup salsa
    1 package Mexican seasoning
    1 can whole-kernel corn (15 oz.)
    1 bag spinach
    ½–1 pound shredded chicken

Bring broth and salsa to a boil. Add remaining ingredients and reduce to a simmer. Top with low-fat cheese.

Makes four servings at approximately 150 calories per serving.

❖ Quick Veggie Logic

Roasted Zucchini and Squash

Preheat oven to 450 degrees. Cut zucchini lengthwise and brush with ½ teaspoon of olive oil. Season with garlic salt and black pepper. Roast in oven for 10 minutes.

Entire serving: 30 calories.

Steamed Broccolini

Purchase broccolini in microwavable bag. Season with your favorite seasoning.

Entire serving: 60 calories.

Spaghetti Squash

Spaghetti squash can be found at your local grocer. Simply follow the directions that come with the spaghetti squash and top with your favorite red sauce.

Makes four servings at approximately 75 calories per serving.

✤ Green Beans . . . Served Hot or Cold!

INGREDIENTS

1½ pounds fresh green beans, trimmed
½ cup olive oil
3 tablespoons balsamic vinegar
½ teaspoon Dijon mustard
1 onion, finely chopped
1 clove garlic, minced
½ cup grated Parmesan cheese
Salt and pepper to taste

This is a great recipe to take to parties! Sprinkle a little salt onto beans and steam them for 6 minutes. Drain well and pat onto paper towel. Blend oil, vinegar, and mustard in a bowl. Add the remaining ingredients, except green beans, to the dressing, pour it over the green beans, and toss lightly.

Makes six servings at approximately 90 calories per serving.

A Healthier Carnivore Treat

I know that a lot of people choose to be vegetarians for moral reasons, which is terriffic. But I also know a lot of people who would find it really hard to not treat their inner carnivore every now and then. Here's how you can transform that sinful steak dinner into a healthier alternative.

First, choose a lean cut of beef. Then take a meat hammer and flatten the steak. Use a palm-size portion and marinate it with a dry rub of your favorite herbs and spices and one tablespoon olive oil. Marinate fresh green beans in a similar marinade—a few teaspoons of dry rub and one table-spoon olive oil. I use a grill pan on my stove at medium heat. Cook steaks to your liking, and for the last few minutes toss the green beans onto the grill pan. Serve.

Now, you may be wondering where the baked potato went. Here's your answer: substitute chicken in place of the steak in this recipe and you can have your baked potato! Spray olive oil on the whole potato and sprinkle with salt and bake it. When it's done, cut it in half and serve it with one to

A GUIDE TO WHAT'S YOUR BEEF

What exactly is a lean cut of beef? When a package says "lean," that means a 3.5-ounce serving contains less than:

- 10 grams total fat
- 4.5 grams saturated fat
- 95 milligrams cholesterol

Some lean cuts of beef are:

- Round steak
- 95 percent lean ground beef
- Chuck shoulder roast
- Arm pot roast
- Shoulder steak
- Strip steak
- Tenderloin steak
- T-bone steak

Extra-Lean Beef
A 3.5-ounce serving of extra-lean beef contains less than:

- 5 grams total fat
- 2 grams saturated fat
- 95 milligrams cholesterol

Some Extra-Lean Cuts of Beef
- Eye of round roast
- Top round steak
- Mock tender steak
- Bottom round roast
- Top sirloin steak

two teaspoons of butter and a seasoning like chives, seasoned salt (not if you're watching sodium intake), or your favorite shaker.

If You Don't Get the Results You Are Looking For

Be patient! Everyone's body is different, and yours may be one that won't respond immediately to the new exercise and nutrition routine. While I want you to be patient and not get frustrated and quit, I don't want you to assume that you are doing everything correctly and your body just isn't responding or the program isn't for you. If you are not losing inches within the first few weeks, you may want to take a look at your food journal—it's very easy to underestimate calories or help yourself to a bigger serving than is allowed in the Nutrition Jump Start. Reduce your intake by 10 percent *or* bump up your cardio!

If you're using my shortcut method to track your calories and you're not seeing the results you'd like, start tracking calories more diligently and using the online resources that are available. You will have to modify and adapt the program to your needs. I know that once you begin exercising, your appetite may increase, and you may unconsciously be consuming more or slightly larger portions than you think.

Are You Getting Enough Calcium?

A mom tells her kids that calcium builds strong teeth and bones. But it does a lot more than that! Calcium helps with muscle contraction and blood clotting. Plus, recent studies show that dairy products actually help promote weight loss.

Women need at least 1,000 milligrams of calcium a day. Women who are over fifty need at least 1,200 milligrams a day. Getting enough calcium can help prevent osteoporosis. Supplementing calcium isn't always necessary if you can add the following foods into your daily intake:

	Serving Size	Calcium (Milligrams, Approximate)
Fruits and Vegetables		
Fruits	1 cup	3
Dairy		
Cheese	1 ounce	200
Cottage cheese	1 cup	50
Pudding	1 cup	150
Milk	1 cup	300
Frozen yogurt	1 cup	200
Low-fat frozen yogurt	1 cup	300
Soy milk	1 cup	10
Cheese pizza	1 slice	250
Breads and Pasta		
Whole-grain bread	1 slice	25
Proteins		
Shrimp	3 ounces	100
Beans	1 cup	50
Peanuts	1 cup	30
Egg	1 egg	30
Tofu	2-by-2-inch piece	100

You can also try calcium-fortified bread, crackers, cereals, sports bars, and juices for added calcium.

On the following page are a couple of recipes to help you get more calcium in your diet without the added calories we usually associate with these dishes.

❖ Reduced-Calorie Broccoli Cheese Soup

1 bag frozen broccoli cuts
2 cups water
2 chicken bouillon cubes
8 ounces reduced-fat cheese (Velveeta works well), cut into cubes
Garlic powder to taste
Salt and pepper to taste

Cook broccoli in water and bouillon cubes until done. Remove half of veggies and mash with fork. Return to pan, add cheese, and heat until melted. Add garlic powder to taste.

Makes four servings at approximately 150 calories per serving.

❖ Reduced-Calorie Macaroni 'n' Cheese

2 cups cooked macaroni
1 cup skim milk or 2 percent milk
8 ounces reduced-fat cheese (Velveeta works well), cut into cubes
Garlic powder to taste
Salt and pepper to taste

Over low heat combine all of the above ingredients. Stir until cheese is melted and pasta is evenly covered.

Makes four servings at approximately 400 calories each.

All of the ideas in this chapter can be applied at any stage in the process: Phase 1, Phase 2, or maintenance. Of course, the sooner you get started, the better off you will be. Unless you're one of those people who would rather run than eat, eating on the run is a fact of life and you can always find a better choice to make that time-crunch meal healthy.

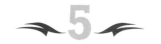

EXERCISE ESSENTIALS

I've already told you that I don't like the word "diet." For me, it brings up images of deprivation and denying ourselves pleasure. When I hear the word, I see myself staring longingly through the window of a Belgian french fry shop in Manhattan, my eyes tearing from the delicious aroma of potatoes dancing in golden oil—only I won't be able to taste the fruits of the chef's efforts! That's torture. For some of you, it may be a bakery or a barbecue that produces similar thoughts and images.

What comes to mind when I say the word "exercise"? I know that some of you may have the same kinds of negative associations with that word that I have with "diet." You may go back to your junior high or high schools days and the tedium of lumbering around a track with a drill sergeant gym teacher harassing you, or you may have visions of dodge balls bouncing off your cranium and you can still feel the sting and see the reddish dimples from where rubber met skin. Even worse, you may shudder when you think of the time you spent slumped over the handlebars of a Schwinn Airdyne Exercise Bike or a StairMaster while some hypercheerful gym rat next to you perkily bounced from one machine to the next, having "just the most super day ever!"

For most of us, exercise is a means to an end. It allows us to feel better, eat more of the foods we tell ourselves we really shouldn't have, and engage in activities that we find fun. Exercise isn't "fun" for most of us, and the words we use to describe our exercise routine reflect that. We went to the gym to "work out." That dreaded W word crops up a lot in conversations about fitness activities.

Let's face facts. Exercise is work. It's work in the way that physicists talk about. It's an expenditure of energy. And that's how we "burn off" excess calories and as a result lose weight. Just like you have to play mental games with yourself when it comes to nutrition, you have to do the same thing when it comes to exercise. If you think about the time you spend working out as time spent burning calories and losing weight instead of time spent mindlessly engaged in repetitive and painful movements, then it may make it easy for you to endure the twenty-five minutes I ask you to do in the Ultimate Six-Week Fitness Plan.

I'd love it if you loved (or grew to love) exercising. I really enjoy moving and get a lot of pleasure from having my body in motion. I find it really freeing to be able to move around and dance as well as being able to perform the controlled movements required by yoga. You may not have had the same kinds of pleasurable experiences I have, but I think that by the time you make it to the end of the Ultimate Six-Week Fitness Plan, you'll have a better appreciation for not just what exercise can do to help you lose weight, but for what your body is capable of doing. I think the human body is a remarkable creation, and giving our bodies a chance to move and to experience the kind of freedom that comes from motion and working in rhythm—whether it's to music or simply the four counts of a jumping jack—releases a whole lot of pent-up tension and anxiety that most of us carry in our bodies.

Being comfortable in your own skin isn't easy, and for some of you, your feelings of self-consciousness have probably gotten in the way of you exercising. All I can say is that you are denying yourself of a lot of pleasure by not exercising. We are human beings living in a body that was meant to move in a variety of ways. Movement is one of the great blessings we have in life, and just as I don't like the word "diet" and all its associations with being deprived and not enjoying life, I'd hate to see you deny yourself the pleasure of movement and not enjoy the enormous blessing of your body in motion.

One of the great pleasures I find in exercise is that I can forget about so many other things when I'm dancing or "working" out. The pressures of home and family and the world just kind of drift off and I'm in my body and not so much in my head. You'd be amazed at how quickly those self-conscious thoughts fade and disappear when you get actively engaged in a

FITTING IT IN

I thought I'd ask some fellow cheerleaders how they find time to fit exercise into their schedule. And although they enjoy exercise, they still have to squeeze it in.

Ashley, a Houston Texans Cheerleader (as well as entrepreneur, cheer coach, and fitness boot camp instructor) shared her insights regarding fitness with me.

LB: What motivates you to stay healthy and fit?

A: Life can't be lived to the fullest if you're not healthy and fit. Being fit gives you a sense of confidence and accomplishment, while being healthy allows you to proactively avoid health issues that can burden you from day to day and sometimes even cause death. I enjoy being healthy and fit and believe that it's a blessing from God that should not be taken for granted. I've lost loved ones to stress and disease and I know that it's my responsibility to take care of myself. This body is the only one that I've got and I plan to do what it takes to keep it in the best shape possible. I've been active my whole life and I'm not sure if I'd know what to do with myself if I ever stopped.

LB: What do you do to stay healthy and fit?

A: Working out is something that I truly enjoy, and I love discovering new and exciting ways to stay fit. I believe that working out should be fun. I guess that's why I love dancing so much; you're getting a workout and you don't even realize it because you're having so much fun.

Not to mention, everything that I do on a day-to-day basis, even outside of Texans cheerleading, requires me to be in tip-top shape. I coach cheer, tumbling, and gymnastics full-time to kids, and it's an absolute must that I stay in shape to be able to keep up with them. I also help instruct fitness boot camps that teach adults and children the importance of staying healthy and fit while kick-starting their exercise program.

LB: How did you mentally and physically prepare for tryouts?

A: I did a combination of things. For starters, I really focused on taking a variety of dance classes to brush up on my dance technique and learn new styles. Being exposed to different styles of dance helped me to become more well rounded so that I'd be ready for anything and less likely to be caught off guard at tryouts. I also went for a three-mile run every morning for about two weeks to lean up. With regards to getting "my look" together, which is also very important, I did research to find out what the Texans wanted and then tried to emulate that and add my own personal touch. By visiting the Texans website, talking to people, and asking lots of questions I was able to go into tryouts more aware and prepared.

> *Tonia is a mother of two, works full-time, and is a five-year veteran of the Tennessee Titans Cheerleaders. I admire her for finding time in her crazy schedule to work out. So I asked her how she does it!*
>
> T: I like to "make the most of my time." I used to teach aerobics and I would get up at 4:30 a.m. to work out. If I don't get a chance in the morning, I work out between work (4:30 p.m.) and practice (7:45 p.m.). I love using Sundays to work out and sometimes Saturdays.
>
> We practice a lot, especially during the summer. But I add running and toning two to three times a week. I do thirty minutes of running and thirty minutes of abs, inner/outer thigh toning, and arms. I believe my workouts should be hard, and I push myself.

physical activity. For a lot of the exercises you're going to be doing, I'll ask that you focus on your body, your breathing, and what each of your muscles is doing. Let the body do its thing and trust that its being in motion will set in motion all of the chemical processes that will produce the kind of weight loss and body sculpting you are looking for.

I know it's a lot to ask you to trust without solid information to back up my request for a leap of faith. For that reason, in the pages that follow, I'm going to give you some basic and some advanced information about the exercise component of fitness and the concepts that underlie my Ultimate Six-Week Fitness Plan. Consider this a brief warm-up phase before we get into the specifics of the exercises themselves.

Getting in the Zone

Researchers have learned that there is a specific level of effort/exertion that we enter into during activity, which forces the body to go to its reserves of fat in order to find the energy it needs to fuel our muscles to perform that activity. The centerpiece of my program is helping you to enter into that "fat-burning zone" as quickly and efficiently as possible. Each workout I've created will allow you to burn 300 calories in thirty minutes. Think of it. For every minute you will be exercising, you will be burning 10 calories. Let's put that in a little more perspective. Remember when I said that it would take a reduction in intake and a burning of excess calories equal to 3,500 in order to lose a pound? Well, I'll let you do the math, but the exercise portion alone of the Ultimate Six-Week Fitness Plan will produce the desired results I've said they will.

How will you get into that fat-burning zone? I've used the term "interval training" before, so it's about time I gave you the specifics of what I mean. During every workout session in the Ultimate Six-Week Fitness Plan, I will lead you through three zones. Because you'll be moving through specific zones that vary the level of intensity at which your body will be working (and therefore your heart will be working at different rates), we call this "zone interval training." These three zones are:

Zone 1: Warm-up interval: Provides toning benefits and a little recovery between Zones 2 and 3.
Zone 2: Aerobic interval: Provides low-intensity fat-burning and toning benefits.
Zone 3: Cardiovascular interval: Provides the highest rate of fat burning.

Every time you exercise following my plan, you will be moving into and out of these three zones. Not only will you be burning excess calories and reducing the amount of fat you carry on your body, you will be boosting your metabolic rate so that even when you're not actively involved in exercise, your body will be burning more calories than before! Along with that, you will be increasing your level of endurance, in addition to toning and strengthening your muscles.

Why Interval Training?

Common sense would tell you that the more intensely you work out and the more effort you exert, the more calories you would burn. Well, that's kind of true, but common sense would also tell you that it is really, really hard to keep up that kind of maximum effort for any length of time. What research has taught us is that the most effective means of fat burning is to go into and out of phases of intense effort. This will optimize the efficiency of the time you spend exercising and produce the kinds of results you really want—shedding excess fat tissue to reveal your fabulous body!

You can apply interval training concepts to any kind of activity you do.

If you are a walker, you will greatly improve the benefits of your walk if you alter the speed/intensity with which you walk. By mixing in bursts of speed with your usual pace, you will get more out of your workout even if you don't increase the amount of total time you walk.

Coaches for elite runners have known this for years, and only in the last few years has the concept really filtered down into the rest of the mainstream health and fitness community. I told you about my marathon-running experience. Well, most of my workouts were run at the same pace—I just ran a longer distance on certain days to work up to the twenty-six miles. If I had really wanted to meet my marathon goal of four hours and thirty minutes, I should have been spending some of those days running shorter distances much faster than my marathon pace. I didn't really know this at the time, but I realize now that doing interval training on the track, even running sprints as short as 200 yards, would have really helped me run the more than 46,000 yards in a marathon.

Yep, shorter and more intense is better for you in lots of ways and in lots of various activities.

EASY ON THE MAYO

Interval training has become such an accepted part of the fitness world, but news of its benefits has also spread into the mainstream health community. The Mayo Clinic, one of the premier hospitals in the country, posted these benefits of interval training on its website:

- You'll burn more calories. The more vigorously you exercise, the more calories you'll burn—even if you increase intensity for just a few minutes at a time.
- You'll improve your aerobic capacity. As your cardiovascular fitness improves, you'll be able to exercise longer or with more intensity. Imagine finishing your sixty-minute walk in forty-five minutes—or the additional calories you'll burn by keeping up the pace for the full sixty minutes.
- You'll keep boredom at bay. Turning up your intensity in short intervals can add variety to your exercise routine.
- You don't need special equipment. You can simply modify your current routine.

(Source: www.mayoclinic.com/health/interval-training/SM00110)

Compound Exercises

I'm all about efficiency and multitasking. I know you don't have hours a day to work out. That's why you'll only be exercising for thirty minutes five times a week. How can you get results when you used to spend up to an hour or an hour and a half every day in the gym? It's easy. Each exercise in my plan is a compound exercise. This means that instead of just targeting one of the major muscle groups, they target at least two and most often more of the major groups on your body. So by doing fewer exercises you can still target all of the areas of your body that need work.

Many of the exercises focus on what is known as your body's core. While there have been a lot of fads in the diet industry, there have been an equal number of fads in the exercise world. One "fad" that won't go away, because it is such a sound principle, is the focus on your core muscles as a true means to achieve fitness. Your core is essentially the center of your body—more specifically, your abdominal muscles. For years people who were serious about fitness spent a lot of time out on their limbs! They would train their legs and their arms. A lot of men, especially, would put such an emphasis on developing a strong (and large) chest and shoulder area. Well, for most people, those muscle groups are more about show and not about go. Sure, who doesn't admire a well-developed and well-toned set of arms? Who doesn't want to look good in a sleeveless dress with tight "guns" instead of sagging hammocks out there for everyone to see?

I have no problem with wanting to have that kind of fitness on your limbs. But that's the icing on the cake and not the cake itself. Unless you really work on your core muscles, you will not be fit. In Pilates, a type of yoga that had been around for years before the concept of core training caught on, the core is also referred to as the "powerhouse." The muscles of the hips, butt, stomach, and lower back truly are the muscles that power us through our day. They are among the largest and often the most neglected muscles.

Why neglected? Well, because we use them all the time to walk, to sit up, and to stand, they are engaged a lot of the time, so we don't often think that they need to be strengthened or worked on. The truth is, because we use them so much, we do need to strengthen them and train them. That sounds kind of odd, but remember what I said earlier about the body being so naturally adaptable. It will try to do things as easily and effortlessly as possible. How many people do you know who get in an elevator or engage in a conversation in a hallway and immediately lean against a wall? Or who, standing in a coworker's doorway to chat, lean against the door's frame? We're unconsciously giving those core muscles, which are used so often, a break.

And how do you think those core muscles come into play when it comes to posture? How many slumped and stooped people do you see every day? Take note sometime of how people hold their bodies. How many of them really have good posture? The reason they don't have good posture, and the reason you may not have good posture, is because the core muscles aren't strong enough.

We often store our excess fat in these areas, too, because these are the areas of our body (hips, butt, and thighs in women and the stomach area in men) that get the least use. So if you want to lose weight and have a fitter, more toned body, you really need to focus on your core. In particular, I'm going to have you focus on your abdominal muscles. While you may not have a rippling six-pack by the time you complete your six-week program, you will have stronger abdominal muscles. You'll find yourself standing taller as a result and looking leaner.

Core 101—An Introduction

Because working your core muscles is so important to overall fitness, even before you get into the fat-burning and cardio target zones I explore with you later in this chapter, I want you to start with these three core exercises today. They take no more than a few moments to learn and to do, and you will immediately feel the benefits. Beginning with these today will also help you do the series of techniques called Ab 5 correctly later on. In my experience, almost 90 percent of women do a crunch wrong and therefore get no benefit from doing core exercises. If you are putting the time in, I would like you to do them right and see results quickly!

Using the transverse abdominis muscle is a big part of my core workout technique. This is a thick layer of muscle that runs from just below your chest down along your stomach to your pelvis on the left and right sides of your body. It wraps around the torso at the waist, and the muscle fibers run horizontally, similar to a corset or a weight belt. This muscle doesn't help move the spine or the pelvis, but it does help with respiration and breathing. It helps you to push air from your lungs, stabilizes the spine, and helps compress the internal organs. These muscles, one on each side, are your true core muscles, and strengthening them will give you power and tone your entire body.

CRUNCH TIME!

For those of you who aren't familiar with a crunch, it is a variation on what you used to do in gym class in school—the sit-up. Because so many of us want to lose the excess around our middles, crunches have become one of the most popular forms of exercise. In my program, you will do many variations of the boring, traditional crunch. But you will need to learn the basics. I can't stress enough how important it is to learn how to do a crunch *properly*. If you don't do it properly you will have a hard time training the deep abdominal muscles, which create a flat stomach. Traditional ab work tends to concentrate on working the rectus abdominis (or your six-pack), which can overdevelop your abdomen. So learn the basics first; then I will ask you to do a lot of variations on the basic crunch with twists, standing, and reversals to work your entire core.

Here's a typical explanation of how to do this simple exercise:

Beginning Phase:

- Lie faceup on a soft surface, bend your knees, and bring your feet close to your butt.
- Fold your arms across your chest, or place your hands behind your head, and tuck your chin into your chest.

Upward Movement:

- Lift with abdominal muscles the upper body toward thighs while keeping the lower back on the floor.

Downward Movement:

- Lower shoulders and upper body slowly and with control.

That's a typical explanation and it's also a *bad* explanation, but it helps to explain why 90 percent of the women I see doing crunches do them wrong. So, what's wrong with this explanation? First, you should *not* tuck your chin into your chest. Lowering your chin to your chest is cheating! It makes it much easier to do the exercise because you are using muscles other than your weak abdominals! Instead lower your eyes to focus on your navel.

Second, this explanation makes no mention of the most important concept of all—in order to fully engage your abdominals, and in particular your transverse abdominis, you have to pull your belly button in toward your spine. This engages the transverse abs, and also works on the other muscles that run along your spine.

Pulling your belly button toward your spine is *not* the same thing as sucking in your gut. What do you do when you suck in your gut? You hold your breath. You don't want to do that. When you are lying on your back and you suck in your gut you hold your breath and what else happens? Try it and find out.

That's right. Your chest rises. That's not what you're trying to do. You want the chest to be still when you pull (not suck in) your abdominal muscles toward your spine. When you are lying on your back, think about someone putting their foot on your belly and pressing it down toward the floor. You can still breathe normally (and that's why your chest can rise and fall), but you aren't holding your expanded chest still.

I will reinforce this important technique later on, but when it comes down to crunch time, think *pull down* and not *suck in*.

Most exercises that work the abs work the smaller abdominal muscles that make up what you see as the so-called six-pack. Six-packs are great, but they really aren't the true core muscles, and the typical crunch that people perform only works those superficial (close to the surface) muscles. We want to work on the deeper abdominal muscles, and that's what the transverse abdominis is—it's the deep abdominal wall. How do you know where those muscles are?

When you "suck in" to put on your skinny jeans, you are engaging the transverse abs. Think about how slim your tummy can get by using your transverse abs while exercising. It is much easier said than done, and before doing the Ab 5 series described in chapters 7 and 8 I would like you to do these simple exercises (and do them all day long) until they become a habit.

1. Find your transverse abdominis. Lie on your back with your knees bent. Breathe in, then exhale and draw your lower abdomen toward the spine. Think hip bones to rib cage. Hold the muscle contraction for 10 seconds, but don't hold your breath. Do not squeeze your butt muscles or your thighs. Repeat ten times.

Find your transverse abdominis.

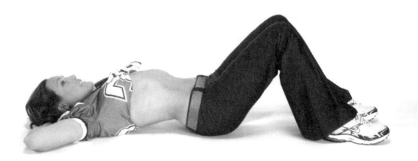

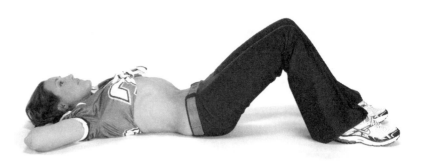

2. Abdominal bracing. Lie on your back with knees bent. Keep your lower back on the ground as you raise your right arm above your head. Then exhale and kick your left leg out. Now switch and raise the left arm over your head. Then kick your right leg out. Throughout the exercise, keep your lower back on the ground and pull your navel toward your spine. Repeat ten times, alternating sides.

Abdominal bracing.

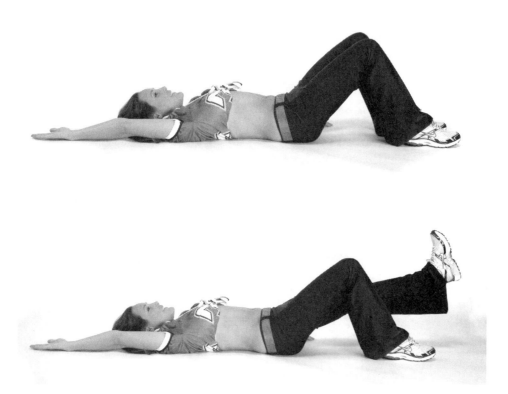

3. Transverse exercise. Place one hand on your belly and perform a regular crunch. If you noticed your belly pooching out as you do this you are not using your transverse abs. Now apply the first technique above as you do your crunch. Your stomach should stay flat as you perform the crunch. Repeat ten times.

You can practice pulling your navel toward your spine anywhere and at any time. I said "practice" but what you'd really be doing is exercising those other abdominals. In fact, as I'm sitting here right now typing, I'm pulling my navel in toward my spine, keeping my chest still while breathing through my nose, holding for a count of ten, and then releasing. I repeat this ten times. You can do this while sitting at your desk at work, while driving (do as many ten-second repetitions as you can while stopped at a red light), while watching television, while reading, or any time and place you find convenient. Start today to jump-start your Jump Start!

Transverse exercise.

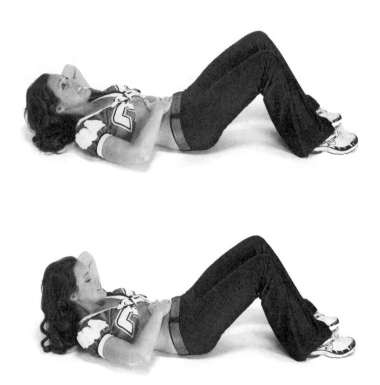

Understanding the Three Zone Intervals

Before you begin any kind of physical activity, it is a good idea to get your muscles loose and relaxed. You don't want to put too much stress and strain on a tight muscle too soon. If you do, you could easily strain or even tear the muscle tissue. Not only are those injuries painful (and easily avoidable), they will prevent you from working out. That will just put you back on the up-and-down roller coaster. When you begin each workout session, you should only feel a slight increase in rate of respiration (the number of breaths you take) and your heart rate (the number of times your heart beats in a given time period). You do not want to exercise at your maximum heart rate (MHR), which is how many times your heart beats during all-out exertion. Instead, it is best to stay between 60 to 90 percent of your target heart rate. Rather than using the Karvonen method to find your target heart rate (THR) I've simplified it into 3 zones. But if you are interested in finding your THR, you can use an online calculator.

In Zone 1, the warm-up range, you will feel that your heart rate has gone up, but it won't feel as though your heart is about to jump out of your chest. You'll feel the effort, but you should still be able to carry on a normal conversation.

Zone 1 is designed to help you warm up and to tone your muscles. A toned muscle is one with clear defining boundaries—you know where your biceps begins and ends. What makes those boundaries visible? An increase in muscle mass (lean body tissue) and a decrease in the amount of fat surrounding that muscle. To tone your muscles you will either use your own body weight or additional free weights to increase the load on the muscle. The only way to build muscle is to increase the load you place on them. I know that some women don't like the muscular look. Don't worry, with my program you won't approach the kind of intensity and loading of muscles that would produce bodybuilder-type muscles. You would have to work out for hours each day doing very specific and very strenuous weight training in order to achieve that look. You don't have enough testosterone in your body to do much else besides tone unless you really dedicated yourself to it.

Zone 1 also gives you an active recovery period before Zone 2 and after Zone 3 and their more intense levels of effort. Why "active recovery"? Because you want to keep your heart rate somewhat elevated over your resting heart rate. So Zone 1 is an "easier" exercise to do in between those more intense periods.

After you warm up, you will move into the more challenging Zone 2, where you'll burn most of your calories. This is the ideal calorie-burning range, and it is where you will spend most of your time while exercising. The exertion it takes to get into this zone varies with people's fitness levels, but you are in Zone 2 when you are at around 65 percent of your maximum heart rate. You will be breathing harder while toning your muscles. And Zone 3 is the most challenging of them all, working at about 85 percent of your maximum heart rate. It will challenge your cardiovascular system, burn the most calories, and have you breathing hard. All three zones will challenge your aerobic and anaerobic levels, mostly aerobic.

"AEROBIC" DEFINED

When I use the word "aerobic" you probably have visions of leotards and leg warmers dancing through your mind. In the 1980s aerobic excercise became all the rage, and Olivia Newton-John and Jane Fonda became as famous for their contributions to fitness as they did for their accomplishments in music and film. But in fact, the word "aerobic" literally means "with oxygen."

Of course, we are always "with oxygen" so I'll explain the term a bit further. Aerobic, as it applies to exercise, means that a rhythmic activity or movement overloads your heart and lungs so that they have to work harder to keep your muscles fueled with oxygen. What separates the aerobic from the anaerobic is the amount of time and the degree to which your heart rate rises. Aerobic exercise is any activity that increases your heart rate for a period of time, long enough to improve your cardiovascular fitness. All the exercise routines in my Ultimate Six-Week Fitness Plan are aerobic activity. An easy way to think of aerobic activities is that they are the ones that make you huff and puff! You'll know when you are in your target zone because your heart rate will climb and your respiration rate will increase. We also call activities and workouts that improve your cardiovascular system "cardio" work. In this book, I will refer to aerobic exercise when I'm referring to lower-intensity work and to cardio work when I'm talking about high-intensity, real huff-and-puff intervals.

To determine whether or not you are in the right zone, I'm going to give you a very useful method called the "perceived exertion" scale. That's a mouthful, but what it basically means is that you determine how hard you feel you're working when involved in an exercise activity. (There's a few of these scales out there, and they may use different terms and comparisons, but they are all doing essentially the same thing.) Instead of taking your pulse, you simply determine how you're feeling. You compare that to how you feel while resting and how you feel while doing other activities.

LINDSAY'S "PERCEIVED EXERTION" SCALE

Some perceived exertion scales go from 1 to 20, but I prefer to only use from 1 to 10. What you are rating is how your heart feels when you are doing each of the activities on the following page. If you've done each of these things before, simply recall how they felt. If you haven't done them, then you can perform the activity and note how you feel when doing each.

ZONE 1 RANGE

1 = Walking briskly
2 = Feeling you get when rushing out the door
3 = End of a dance class warm-up
4 = Low dance kicks for a few minutes

When you are in Zone 1, the hardest you should feel you are working is what you would feel like if you were doing those low dance kicks. When you are in Zone 1 you are either in the "warming up" phase or in the "active recovery" phase. What is "active recovery"? That's when you are slowing the pace to allow your heart rate to slow. You aren't stopping movement completely, but you are taking it down a few notches so that your heart and respiration rates slow.

ZONE 2 RANGE

5 = Jogging (or speed walking) one mile for physical fitness class
6 = It's getting hard to sing and dance at the same time
7 = Just finishing a fast hip-hop dance

When you are in Zone 2, the aerobic interval, your heart should be beating like it would if you were doing one of the activities listed here. This is where you will spend most of your time during my workouts. How well you can breathe to carry on a conversation is a useful measure of your exertion level. In this zone, you should still be able to speak while you do the exercise. It may not be perfectly easy for you to speak, but you should still be able to do it without taking in huge gulps of air. Remember, this zone is the lower-intensity fat-burning zone.

ZONE 3 RANGE

8 = Breathing hard, as you would in a kick line
9 = Performing high kicks for two minutes

10 = Running seventy yards with a touchdown pass, with the defense trailing you

When you are in Zone 3 you are at your "fitness threshold." Push any harder and you will crash through the door into oxygen debt and maxing out your heart rate. You don't want to cross that line, but you certainly want to be able to see the line and nudge your toe up against it. This is the high-intensity fat-burning zone that you will move into and out of more quickly than the steadier effort of Zone 2.

MOVING THROUGH THE ZONES

Each zone has its specific benefits, but all of them will help your body to burn calories more efficiently. As a result, your fitness threshold will go up. You will be able to do more and for longer periods of time before you feel like you can't go on. That also means that you will be able to burn more calories. That's the kind of exercise cycle you will be glad to engage in! The American College of Sports Medicine (ACSM) recommends that you engage in at least twenty to sixty minutes of aerobic activity at least three times a week. That means that you should be working at 65–90 percent of your maximum heart rate or getting into and staying at Zone 2 for that amount of time. I've based my ultimate plan on these recommendations, and if you follow it, you will be easily achieving what the experts recommend.

What I ask you to do is to get to these levels as you move through each of the zones. If you want to count heartbeats, that means that you should be at these levels:

Zone 1 = 60–70 percent of your target heart rate
Zone 2 = 70–80 percent of your target heart rate
Zone 3 = 80–90 percent of your target heart rate

If you are using my "perceived exertion" scale, then that means:

Zone 1 = 1 to 4 (Okay! I can do this.)
Zone 2 = 5 to 7 (Whew! This is getting tougher.)
Zone 3 = 8 to 10 (Wow! I don't know how long I can keep this up.)

If you ever get to a point when that *Wow!* turns to *Oww!* you should slow down gradually and then stop. If it's a real *Zowww!* then stop immediately. "No pain no gain" is not a good motto to have. Pain is your friend, because pain will tell you that something is not right. Listen to what she's saying. Learn the difference between discomfort/effort and pain. Exercise should be hard but it shouldn't truly be painful. (Although I've often said "Ow!" at the end of a game after cheering in high-heeled boots for four hours!)

~ 6 ~

A FEW THINGS YOU SHOULD KNOW AND

A FEW MYTHS YOU SHOULD FORGET

After the first fifteen minutes of a football game, the teams take a short break. The TV broadcast goes to commercial, and most home viewers make a trek to the bathroom or to the kitchen to get more food and beverages. While all of you are busy doing that, the women on the cheerleading squad go to work. These are the moments we worked so hard for in the off season and during the week of practice leading up to the game. While the fans in the stands appreciated our efforts, I'm not sure how visible our contribution was to everyone watching the game from the comfort of their family room.

People often asked if we knew when we were going to be on camera. The answer is yes and no. It's hard to ignore the presence of television cameras at the game, particularly when it's a hand-held one just a few inches away from you! The thing is, however, you're so into the flow of the game that you don't really think about the cameras being there at all. When we performed, regardless of whether the camera was on us or not, we had to give 100 percent of our effort and focus. We never really knew for sure when the camera lens was focused directly on one of us and whether that shot was the one the director was choosing to show the audience.

In some ways, that's kind of what it's like with diet and exercise programs. Some of the time, people will notice the change in your shape, your attitude, etc. What they don't see is all the hard work and effort you put into producing those results. The other thing is, you have to keep putting out the effort even if you don't think that anyone is watching you or commenting on the changes you notice. I know that a lot of the time you will be working out alone. Who's going to notice if you only do twenty crunches instead of twenty-five? Who's going to notice if you have that second slice of devil's food cake?

The truth is, *you will*. Just like we cheerleaders have to give it our all no matter who or what had an eye trained on us, you have to take that same level of commitment to your diet and exercise routines. Your new habits will help you eliminate the excess calories that turn to fat. And as we've seen, some very small daily changes can lead to losing weight and reducing the amount of unhealthy and unsightly fat on your body. The great thing is, you can do these things starting today! Add your exercises consistently and you will lose approximately one to two pounds per week. Even better, you will lose weight the healthy way and keep the weight off.

Before we get into more specifics, I want to take advantage of this brief time out to recap some key concepts and to put to rest some myths about diet and exercise that you may be carrying around. Here are the five things you need to do in order to improve your health.

Turn Up the Volume!

Like I mentioned in our discussion of nutrition, it is so important to eat high-volume foods and avoid empty ones. High-volume foods contain a lot of fiber and water to keep you satisfied and provide you with a rich mix of nutrients and vitamins. Among the high-volume foods you should be making a regular part of your meal planning are lean proteins, vegetables, fruits, soups, whole grains, and salads. Soup is one of my favorite high-volume foods. Soups are packed with nutrients and so filling (just make sure you keep an eye on the sodium content if buying a canned soup!). I frequently don't have a lot of time to cook, but I can make a big pot of soup and then freeze lunch-size portions for quick meals later.

FAT-BURNING SUPERFOODS

A lot has been written recently about so-called superfoods. You know, the ones that (if you believe all the hype) you eat and they somehow magically work in your system to burn fat off your body. Well, the truth is that no food is a superfood in that sense. Nothing you can eat will magically burn fat from your body! Your body will burn the calories contained in the food, but those foods won't go on to set off some kind of metabolic chain reaction that will send cellular flamethrowers to your hips and thighs to get rid of unwanted fat deposits there.

Sorry for that bit of bad news.

High-volume foods, in my mind, are the fat-burning superfoods. These foods are full of fiber, water, and other nutrients. They make you feel full faster and therefore you consume fewer calories of them. When you consume fewer calories and increase the amount of calories you're burning, your body eventually goes to your fat stores to get you the energy you need. Ideally, we want your fat stores to be like your local convenience store, where you go to pick up a couple of essentials on an as-needed basis. Unfortunately, for too many of us, our fat stores are more like giant supermarkets or price clubs where we stock too much of our reserves.

High-volume foods will have your body shopping at those fat stores, eventually reducing their stock to convenience store–size portions.

What are some other high-volume foods? Think greens. Salad greens—minus the cheese and fatty dressings, etc.—are a great source of fiber, water, and minerals. There are so many more varieties of lettuce available to us today that the usual run-of-the-mill iceberg variety shouldn't have to dominate your salad intake (not to mention that iceberg lettuce isn't nearly as rich in nutrients). They range in flavors from buttery (like Boston) to spicy (like arugula) and have the same caloric value as the tried-and-true iceberg.

Beans are another high-volume food that will enable you to tap into your fat reserves. As an added plus, they are a great source of protein. Studies have shown that since protein takes longer to break down chemically, it stays with you longer and keeps you feeling fuller longer. That's a win-win situation.

Green tea. It's going to take a lot more study to convince me that green tea actually stimulates your body to burn more calories. But it is a great after-dinner treat to ward off the calories! And although it has many other great qualities, like lowering cholesterol, suppressing your appetite, and aiding in digestion, it does not burn fat. No foods do, these high-volume foods are simply healthy options.

> **Some Other Great High-Volume Foods**
>
> Tea and coffee (careful with the caffeine)
> Low-fat cottage cheese
> Chicken, shrimp, salmon
> Soup, especially broth-based soups like vegetable and chicken noodle
> Barley
> Whole-grain products like oatmeal and whole-wheat pasta
> Beans
> Apples, berries, melons

Here's a "loud" (high volume—get it?) quiz for you:

4 cups of popcorn vs. 2 chocolates
1 cup of grapes vs. 4 tortilla chips
1 dozen shrimp vs. 2 bites of steak

The answer is, of course, that each of the items listed first is the high-volume choice. It's nice to know that you can eat more of some things and have them be better for you and satisfy you more fully than others!

A way to cut down on the portions of your main meals is by healthy snacking. I know a lot of women who believe that if they cut out the snacks, they're going to manage their weight better. I'm a bit of a believer in the "eat less more frequently" principle. In other words, consume fewer calories at any one time but eat more times during the course of the day. Snacks help to take the edge off your hunger and will keep you from feeling deprived. When you feel deprived, you often fall to the temptation of splurging. Avoid the splurge and eat frugally and frequently.

Here are some high-volume snacks you can use to get a lasting energy boost and to take a bite out of your hunger:

- 2–3 ounces of peanut butter with a piece of fruit. Apples, pears, and bananas are especially tasty with peanut butter!
- 6 cups of light popcorn (season with cheese sprinkles for cheddar corn)

- 6 strawberries dipped in low-fat pudding
- 1 handful of almonds
- 12 whole-grain crackers with low-fat cheese
- 2 pieces of whole-grain bread with 1 tablespoon of peanut butter
- Cut-up vegetables with hummus
- Turkey sandwich
- 1 cup broth-based soup
- Small salad with veggies
- Dozen shrimp

Again, I know how busy your week is, so prepare these snacks ahead of time (maybe while that soup is simmering on the stove) so that you don't have an excuse later on for grabbing the more convenient candy bar, cookies, chips, sodas, etc. Those empty-calorie snacks (high in calories, low in nutrients) may satisfy a craving, but they don't satisfy your hunger, and you'll find yourself consuming more and more. Don't get caught in that loop.

HOW TO GET MORE HIGH-VOLUME FRUITS AND VEGGIES INTO YOUR DAY

1. Keep a fruit bowl on the kitchen table. When you see the fruit you will eat it, and possibly come to crave it!
2. Add vegetables to any pasta dish.
3. Base your meal around vegetables, not protein. Fill half your plate with vegetables.
4. Make leftover vegetables by cooking twice as much as you need at any meal.
5. Add fruit to cereal and oatmeal, or use as a dessert at dinner.
6. Snack on raw veggies.
7. Eat veggie pizza instead of pepperoni or sausage.
8. Mix berries, yogurt, and ice for a fruit smoothie. It's easy to get all servings of fruit this way!
9. Use frozen vegetables and fruits. They are packaged at their ripest time.

I know some people love to have a laid-back start to their mornings. Nutritionists will tell you that you should eat your breakfast as close as possible to the time you wake up and preferably no later than one to three hours after you get out of bed. Why? First of all, breakfast is breaking the fast you've undergone by not eating for the hours leading up to—and including—your sleep. Your blood sugar is low and in order to even it out, you should eat as soon as possible. If you don't, you set up another of those calorie splurge cycles—hunger will get to you, you will need a quick fix, the quick fix won't satisfy you, and you will eat more than you really need because those empty calories are burned so quickly. That sets you up for a bad eating day.

✤ Breakfast Burritos

INGREDIENTS
- ⅓ pound turkey sausage
- 12 egg whites or egg substitute
- 1 green pepper
- 1 red pepper
- 1 teaspoon olive oil
- 6 whole-wheat tortillas
- 4 ounces low-fat cheese

Make these ahead of time for breakfast on the go! Cook turkey sausage in skillet, drain, and set aside. Then scramble egg whites or egg substitute in the same skillet; set aside. Sauté green and red peppers in 1 teaspoon olive oil. Combine egg whites, turkey sausage, and peppers. Place one-sixth of mixture on 1 whole-wheat tortilla and sprinkle a little bit of cheese on top. Wrap tortilla into a burrito. Wrap individually in plastic wrap and freeze or refrigerate.

❖ Sweet Wraps

INGREDIENTS

1 whole-wheat tortilla
½ apple, sliced
½ teaspoon sugar
dash of cinnamon

Place apple on the tortilla and sprinkle with the sugar and cinnamon. Wrap and heat for 30 seconds.

❖ English Muffin Melt

INGREDIENTS

1 whole-grain English muffin
2 tomato slices
1 slice low-fat cheese, divided into two pieces

Split open English muffin. On each half place 1 tomato slice and a half slice of cheese. Brown under a broiler until cheese is melted.

You should also make sure that your breakfast contains both fiber and calcium. You can do this by eating fruit and adding milk or yogurt or other dairy to it. A good wholesome start to your day could include oatmeal and

---

I DON'T HAVE TIME FOR BREAKFAST!

- Fruit is easy for a quick bite. After you purchase fruit from the grocery store, wash and put it in easy-to-grab containers.
- Drinkable yogurt is good for you and easy to drink on the go!
- A whole-wheat English muffin with peanut butter travels well.
- Make smoothies ahead of time with fruit, ice, milk, and yogurt.
- Grab a protein bar with at least five grams of fiber.
- Prepare eggs, green peppers, tomatoes, and low-fat cheese in whole-wheat tortillas. Freeze and pop in the microwave for a quick meal.

---

fruit, or a whole-wheat English muffin with 2 percent low-fat melted cheese on it. Our mothers were right when they talked about food "sticking to our ribs." Oatmeal takes a long time to digest, gives you that feeling of being "full" longer, and provides you with a steady stream of nutrients to avoid the peaks and valleys that have you craving those empty sugary quick fixes.

Stay Hydrated

Our lean muscle, blood, and brain tissue are each made up of more than 70 percent water. Every system in our body needs water. As I stated before, unfortunately, most of us don't drink enough water each day. Every day our bodies lose eight to twelve cups of water just carrying away waste and cooling us, among other things. At minimum those eight to twelve cups need to be replaced.

Helpful hint: When I'm trying to lose a few pounds, I will drink one glass of water before a meal and another during the meal to make myself feel fuller.

Eat Less More Frequently

To keep up your energy, you need to consume some calories every few hours. Again, the point here is to avoid the peaks and valleys that have you grabbing a quick and unhealthy sugar fix. Eating three meals a day with one to two snacks in between is ideal. Keep in mind the number of calories you need to consume to maintain your BMR, and don't exceed that amount. If you can eat every few hours, and add in even a minimal amount of daily exercise, you will boost your metabolism and be on your way to burning more calories regularly.

Let's recap. Here are the five things you can do every day to make yourself healthier and a better eater.

1. Eat high-volume foods!
2. Learn and use the proper method to determine serving size.
3. Eat breakfast within three hours of waking up.
4. Drink the right amount of water.
5. Eat less at one time, but eat more often.

- **Drink while exercising.** This is especially true if you are pregnant. To prevent dehydration while exercising you must replace water at a faster rate. I recommend at least two cups before and after exercise. You should also drink about one cup every fifteen minutes during exercise.
- **Don't underestimate water.** Water carries away waste, transports nutrients, regulates body temperature, helps detoxify your system, and cushions the body from injury. Every day you lose an average of eight to twelve cups of water that need replacing.
- **Watch for dehydration.** Mild dehydration can lead to lethargy and constipation. Dehydration symptoms include minor headaches, loss of appetite, and dizziness.
- **Drink before you're thirsty.** Many experts believe that if you wait until you are thirsty, you are already slightly dehydrated.
- **Too much water?** If you notice unexplained increases in thirst and urination, consult your health-care provider. These can be symptoms of diseases such as diabetes. Hyponatremia is a condition in which the body gets too much water. This can occur in marathon runners and infants if too much water is consumed in a small amount of time.
- **Exercise sessions of ninety-plus minutes require sports drinks.** If you happen to be a marathon runner or triathlete, it's recommended that you drink sports drinks instead of water. These beverages contain electrolytes (like sodium and potassium) to enhance fluid absorption and carbohydrates to boost energy.
- **Ways to drink more water.** Tea, milk, lemonade, and juices are made up of mostly water. You can also get water from sources like salad, veggies, and fruits. Caffeine can somewhat dehydrate you, so drink a glass of water for every cup of caffeinated beverage.

Setting the Record Straight: Workout and Diet Myths

■ **A snack-size bag of crackers is just as healthy as an apple.**

In general, you should avoid eating anything boxed or bagged. First of all, they are not filling. Second, they frequently contain the dreaded bad fat: hydrogenated oil. That processed oil may increase the product's shelf life, but end up putting you on the shelf in the long run. Try this experiment. One day go to the snack machine at work and eat the snack-size bag or bar of your choice. The next day, bring an apple and a few ounces of peanut butter from home. Compare how hungry you felt later after eating each. I'm willing to bet the apple and peanut butter stayed with you longer and was more satisfying.

- **Organic foods have fewer calories.**

Wrong. How a product is grown, with natural fertilizers or without pesticides, has no effect on its calorie content. They are generally healthier but not less rich in calories. You can still gain weight eating organic!

- **Brown rice is better for me than white rice.**

Yes, brown rice has more nutrients, but it does contain the same number of calories.

- **Brown sugar is healthier than white sugar.**

Nope. Although the added molasses in brown sugar is quite rich in nutrients, very little of that makes its way into brown sugar, so it is not better for you.

- **You will not lose weight if you eat after seven o'clock at night.**

It doesn't matter when you eat, your body will process the food. The reason why many health and fitness professionals recommend you not eat at night is that women tend to consume a lot of calories at night when they are winding down. It's not a question of when, but how many calories you are consuming.

- **Once I start exercising, I need to consume more food.**

Again, this isn't true. When you exercise, particularly at the beginning of a program, you will need to burn off the excess calories you stored up during your preworkout days. If you start eating more when you begin to exercise, all you're doing is adding more calories to be burned.

- **In order to burn off the calories contained in one cookie, you have to exercise for ten minutes.**

Try *forty* minutes. That's right, it will take nearly three-quarters of an hour of exercise to burn off those calories. Even a relatively small (1 oz.)

cookie made from those refrigerated rolls contains about 125 calories. Most of us underestimate how much work it takes to burn off that large cookie. As a result, we can't lose weight.

■ **Eating certain foods can eliminate fat from specific areas of your body.**

If only that were true! All kinds of books and DVDs make this fantasy seem real, but the truth is that your genetics determine which areas of your body will lose first. My diet and exercise program will help you lose fat from every part of your body, and you can target certain areas with exercise but not with specific foods.

■ **Doing thirty minutes of abdominal work will slim my waistline.**

Maybe, but you must do cardio work as well. There is no such thing as spot-reducing weight loss—your genetics determine where you lose weight at first. But you can spot-train muscles—you can tone certain areas of muscle.

Reality Check

Okay, I've said some of things in different ways before, but let's take a minute to check ourselves back into our room at the Reality Hotel. (Fortunately, there are always rooms available here since we like to trick ourselves into believing so many things that we wish were true!)

Fad diets don't work. Low-carb, no-carb, low-protein, low-fat—it doesn't matter. They get a lot of hype so we think they're effective. Well, they're not. What is effective is cutting the amount of calories you consume or burning more calories. If you've tried other plans and wound up losing and then regaining, that's because fad diets don't work. So let's get real and take a look at a couple of key ideas:

■ Half the battle in losing weight and feeling good is knowing what *not* to do.
■ Most fad diets are essentially low-calorie plans in disguise. Remember: 3,500 calories consumed = one pound of weight gained. If you want to lose a pound, you have to lower your caloric intake and in-

crease your caloric burning. Those diets encouraging you to eat as much of a type of food as you want will only lead you to have a nutritional imbalance that will lead to irritability and low energy.

- Water weight loss versus real weight loss. Want to know why low-carb diets have you losing weight initially? When your body is starved of carbohydrates, you stop refilling the stores of glycogen in your body. Glycogen is like a water magnet. It attracts water. If you don't have a lot of glycogen in your body, you don't have as much water stored in your body. Water weight loss will show up when you step on the scale, and you think, "Hey, this diet is working!" The truth is that it's really not working. You're dehydrated—which makes you irritable and saps your energy—and worse, you're not losing the fat that you want to get rid of!

- There are no magic food combinations. You can't target areas of your body with specific foods, nor is there any scientific basis to support the grapefruit and tuna fish diet somehow putting your body chemistry to work to produce miraculous weight loss numbers.

- Diet fatigue causes more "failures" than any other factor. We want and need variety in our diets. If you eliminate a type of food, you will end up at some point craving it. You will get bored with the low-carb/low-protein fad diet routine. Not only will diet fatigue set in, but real fatigue will as well. If you're not taking in the proper nutrients you'll also lack energy.

I can't even begin to tell you how many clients I tried to persuade to eat healthy and not go on a particular fad diet. Well, about half of them listened; the other half did not. The half that chose the protein-based diet *initially* lost weight. But unfortunately, they all gained the weight back plus additional pounds. And the weight gain was now pure fat!

One of my good friends on the squad chose to go for the protein-based diet before the calendar shoot. The same thing happened. She looked fabulous for the swimsuit calendar but ended up battling a few extra pounds during the season. She kept attempting to eat all protein, but she had cravings just like anybody else. And the protein diet is one you *cannot* stray from or you will gain weight immediately. Not only did she battle a few extra pounds all season, but her energy was zapped. She was usually full of energy—she was a full-time student in addition to cheering so she needed all that energy—but I definitely noticed she was tired all the time. Every practice became a job and a countdown until she could go home.

You don't want to end up like that, especially since in the next chapter, we're getting into the "meat" of the matter. We're going to look at Phase 1—the first three weeks of the Ultimate Six-Week Fitness Plan! On the next page prepare to shed those pounds you thought you'd lost forever with one of those fad diets!

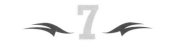

THE ULTIMATE SIX-WEEK FITNESS PLAN

Phase 1— Break Through to New Habits

Okay, the pregame festivities are over and it's nearly game time. I've given you a lot of information to mentally prepare you for what you're about to undertake. Now it's the day of the game and we're going to finally execute the game plan we've been reviewing. If you're anything like me, you're probably anxious to get going. That's how I was when I was cheering. I couldn't wait for game days. I had to develop a typical routine for game time to relieve anxiety and help me stay focused so I could be the cheerleader I wanted to be.

Four hours before game time, my husband would drop me off at the entrance where all Rams employees—players, cheerleaders, coaches, and staff—gained access to the dome. He'd wish me luck and give me a kiss and tell me he'd see me after the game. I also knew I'd get to see him during the game because my family are all huge Rams fans and they attend every home game. As soon as we got into the dome, we'd go through a security check, which involved opening our Rams suitcase to show our pom-poms, outfit for after the game, and the present we'd brought for our "Big Sis" or "Lil Sis." We wore our practice outfits going to the dome and changed into skirts and suits to leave the dome after the game. Of course we carried our boots and game-day uniform, too. Almost all squads wear white boots—so that even the fans in the "nosebleed" section can see our legs when we do our kick lines.

Most days when we practiced, wherever we gathered at the players' practice dome, we made a lot of noise and had to be quieted by one of our coaches, but a lot of game-day Sundays began at 8:00 a.m. so things were pretty quiet. Most of us hadn't fully woken up, and we had a lot on our minds. As soon as we arrived, we went to get our hair and makeup done. We all had our favorite stylist and lined up waiting for our turn with him or her. Sitting in that chair was pretty relaxing, and I think that had a lot to do with how quiet we stayed. While waiting, we could select from a food spread in the middle of the room. Just like at practice, we were also offered some of the same foods the players ate at games. But we always joked about how the team sent us the stuff the players didn't want. We usually had wraps, yogurt, fruit, cereal, crackers, veggies and dip, and we always had these broken cookies—we wondered if someone had tackled the box, but eventually figured out that the broken cookies were to mix with the yogurt! I would usually eat just a little bit—heck, I had to be in a two-piece midriff-exposing uniform in front of 65,000 fans in three hours! Nothing like that to keep you motivated to eat lightly on game days.

Once my makeup and hair were done I went back to my locker to put on my uniform. We had to wear fishnet hose under our skirts, and one of Lindsay's Secrets is that these undergarments had the most unflattering waistband. We usually passed around some scissors to snip the top off the hose, so it didn't look like we all had rolls hanging over the waistband. Another secret? Do you think most cheerleaders have big boobs? Think again! While many of the women could thank nature and genetics, I wasn't one of them. My mom got pretty good at sewing "enhancers" into my outfits!

We zipped up our boots and were required to be on the field exactly forty minutes before a game. It was time to sell calendars for charity and see our fans! Sometimes we got ready an hour or two before the game to collect money for our troops in the area outside where attendees park and tailgate.

Another of Lindsay's Secrets, I must admit, is that after the game I always had my husband stop at Taco Bell (yes, one of my favorite spots) so I could get two bean burritos and some chips. Since I hadn't eaten much all day, even eating that relatively small amount usually put me into a food coma. We would get home and I would nap while he watched more football. Would I ever recommend not eating for most of the day and crashing like I did—heck, no! But it's what I did because it made me feel confident and made me feel I looked good on the field. Our uniforms would reveal even the smallest one-pound weight gain or water weight. So I always watched especially carefully what I ate the day before a game, ate lots of veggies and protein, and drank a ton of water—in other words, I followed my "how to get a flat tummy in one day" plan I told you about in the introduction.

Your In-Season Routine

It was important for me to develop a routine, a kind of road map. That's what these next chapters are all about. Getting you into a routine and providing you with a road map so that you can eliminate distractions and focus on getting the job done. This chapter contains all of the details you need for the first three weeks of the Ultimate Six-Week Fitness Plan. (Chapter 8 contains the details for the final three weeks.)

As I mentioned, I've divided the program into two phases: the three weeks of Phase 1 are designed to jump-start your body and keep your mind engaged. Phase 2 takes the program to the next level, introducing a new set of exercises and meal plans for the last three weeks. Every week of the six-week plan features a different workout, with three days of the Get into Your Fat-Burning Zone method and two days of the Cardio Zone. The other two days are for you to rest! Best of all, each workout can be done in thirty minutes or less.

The result? You're going to increase your metabolism, burn fat, and tone and tighten, and the best part is you're going to find muscles you never knew you had.

THE ROOTS OF THE EXERCISES

Most of the compound exercises I have you do are derived mainly from Pilates or dance methods. In dance you do have to use strength training to improve your endurance, to kick high, and to do leaps and jumps. Some cheerleading squads even do more gymnastic moves, with male cheerleaders helping out with lifts and other stunts. More common exercises like push-ups come at the end of practice because there are not many dance moves that target your chest muscles! As you perform the exercises you will notice you use your core in a majority of them. For example, when you do a triceps kickback, you do it from a position called the Warrior. This works not only the backs of your arms (triceps kickback) but your lower body and helps improve your balance! All dancers need balance! And balance comes from your muscles working in opposition to one another. This push-pull between what are referred to as "antagonistic" muscles is essential for balance. The only way to strengthen those muscles and improve your balance is to do moves that require you to balance yourself, and to do strength training of the individual muscles and muscle groups.

One very common dance move I will have you move into and out of is the plié. It works not only your balance but your inner and outer thighs and core. Dancers perform pliés from different foot positions (1st, 2nd, 3rd, 4th, and 5th). There is a demi plié and a grand plié. You will do both from 1st and 2nd position. To make things easier for you and to eliminate some extra terminology for you to know, I will describe the dance moves rather than use their names, but rest assured, you will be doing many dance-related moves during your workout.

Nutrition Jump Start

I know that for some of you, counting calories is going to be a drag. If that's the case, use the shortcut method I outlined in chapter 4 and note how much of each of the food groups you eat during your first three weeks. I know you have the additional burden of starting a fitness program, and I want this to be easy. If you find that you are losing the kind of weight you want to by following the shortcut plan, you can stick with it in Phase 2. If you find you aren't as successful as you'd hoped to be in Phase 1, then in Phase 2, you can kick things up a notch by actually counting calories according to my guidelines by food group in chapter 4. And even if you get good results in Phase 1 with the shortcut method, you can still switch to the calorie-counting method to see if by refining your calorie tracking you can improve your weight loss.

Starting Is the Hardest Part

I know that the first three weeks of this will probably seem the most challenging, as your body adjusts to a new routine and you consume fewer calories. In terms of the fitness plan, you can expect to experience some soreness. After all, you likely haven't used your muscles or your heart like this before or in a long time, so give yourself some time, have fun, and then we'll change it up again in Phase 2! You're also likely to experience the highest degree of discomfort with the nutrition plan at the beginning, but that, too, will pass with time. Just be patient. Don't beat yourself up or give up if you slip up, and know that after the first twenty-one days, your body will be adjusted and you'll be over that first hump!

HERE'S YOUR SCHEDULE FOR THE ULTIMATE SIX-WEEK FITNESS PLAN
- Monday—Get into Your Fat-Burning Zone*
- Tuesday—Cardio Zone
- Wednesday—Get into Your Fat-Burning Zone*
- Thursday—Cardio Zone
- Friday—Get into Your Fat-Burning Zone*
- Saturday—Rest or workout makeup
- Sunday—Rest or workout makeup

*You can substitute the "10-Minute Workout" (see page 214) on busy days, but try to limit these.

(Note: If you haven't worked out in more than a year, you may want to spend more than one week in each week of the program. Check with your doctor before beginning any exercise program.)

The Routine

The guide that follows is your list of daily exercises for the next three weeks, and the exercises should be performed in the order I present them. I also include a warm-up and cooldown set of exercises for the Get into Your Fat-Burning Zone days. You should do these each time you exercise. And I give you suggested Cardio Zone exercises that include warm-up and cooldown segments.

You can find full descriptions of each exercise, including how to perform them, helpful hints, and two to three photos that make learning them easy. The exercises in the main body of the workout are organized into blocks that contain three exercises—one in each of three zones. You will do six blocks each time in the main portion of your workout. I will add in a new block after Week 1, but I will also delete one, so that you will never do more than six blocks. I always want your workouts to last no more than thirty minutes.

Once you've mastered the exercises, you may find the Quick Reference Guide at the back of the book is all you need. It lists each exercise by name and the order in which you will do them. I also include one photo to remind you of how the exercise is performed. I'd rather have you focused on the exercises than looking at the book for guidance. It will take a bit of time, but eventually you won't have to have the book by your side as you exercise!

General Guidelines

Remember, you're challenging the heart rate in different zones for the most effective workout. How challenging should it be? Remember, you can use either my "perceived exertion" scale or the heart rate method to make sure you work your way into each zone. (See pages 108–110 if you need a refresher.)

- In Zone 1 exercises, you should feel as if you are warming up or recovering. When warming up, your heart rate will be increasing; when recovering it will be going down.
- Zone 2 is your "aerobic" workout, when your breathing gets faster and you begin to substantially get your heart rate up.

■ Zone 3 is the huff-and-puff zone, which is meant to put your heart at its fitness threshold.

Lindsay's "Perceived Exertion" Scale

Zone 1 = 1 to 4 (Okay! I can do this.)
Zone 2 = 5 to 7 (Whew! This is getting tougher.)
Zone 3 = 8 to 10 (Wow! I don't know how long I can keep this up.)

The Heart Rate Method

The Karvonen method factors in resting heart rate (HR_{rest}) to calculate target heart rate (THR):

$$THR = [(MHR - HR_{rest}) \times \text{percent intensity}$$
$$60\%, 70\%, 80\%, \text{ or } 90\%] + HR_{rest}$$

You get your resting heart rate by counting the beats of your heart for 1 minute before getting out of bed. You get your MHR from the following formula (recent evidence from USA researchers) MHR = $206.9 - (0.67 \times \text{age})$.
Record your target heart rate here _____.

Zone 1 = 60–70 percent of your Target Heart Rate	Record your Zone #1 Heart Rate here: _____
Zone 2 = 70–80 percent of your Target Heart Rate	Record your Zone #2 Heart Rate here: _____
Zone 3 = 80–90 percent of your Target Heart Rate	Record your Zone #3 Heart Rate here: _____

Sometimes I'll ask you to move from a standing position to a lying position. If you ever feel your heart is beating too fast, please take a small break before going to the ground.

BREATHING 101

You've probably heard of singers, wind instrument musicians, and actors talking about the importance of breathing through the diaphragm. They do it because it helps them to control the amount of air they are using. Using proper breathing technique is important for any activity or just daily living, but it is especially important that you breathe properly when working out. Consciously using your diaphragm is the most efficient way to breathe. The diaphragm is a large, dome-shaped muscle located at the base of your lungs. Your abdominal muscles help move the diaphragm and give you more power to empty your lungs. When you don't use your diaphragm to breathe properly, air can get trapped in your lungs. That air pushes down on your diaphragm and can flatten the dome shape of the muscle and weaken it. When you don't breathe properly, the neck and muscles have to pitch in and that means the diaphragm is working even less.

Diaphragmatic breathing will help you to:

- Strengthen the diaphragm muscle
- Decrease the work of breathing by slowing your breathing rate
- Decrease oxygen demand
- Use less effort and energy to breathe

Here's how to properly breathe through your diaphragm. It's a simple and natural process (if you fall asleep on your back you can't help but breathe this way) that will soon become second nature.

1. Lie on your back on a flat surface or in bed, with your knees bent and your head supported. (You can use a pillow under your knees to support your legs, if needed.) Place one hand on your upper chest and the other just below your rib cage. This will allow you to feel your diaphragm move as you breathe.
2. Breathe in slowly through your nose so that your stomach moves out against your hand. The hand on your chest should keep as still as possible.
3. Tighten your stomach muscles, letting them fall inward as you exhale through pursed lips. Keep the hand on your upper chest as still as possible.

When you first learn the diaphragmatic breathing technique, it'll be easier for you to follow the instructions lying down. When you get better at it, you can try the diaphragmatic breathing technique while sitting in a chair. Repeat the same steps as above. You can also do this while standing and while exercising. Remember, inhale through the nose and exhale through the mouth.

You'll also find that this breathing technique will help you relax! If you're having trouble sleeping at night, lie on your back and use this technique to inhale deeply for six seconds and exhale thoroughly for six seconds. In no time at all you should relax enough to drift off to sleep!

Repetitions

- Always do twenty repetitions of both Zone 1 and Zone 2 exercises. (You'll need your free weights for some of these.)
- Spend one minute on Zone 3 exercises.
- Do the Ab 5 series at the end of every workout.

Halftime Festivities

You will notice that at the midpoint of every workout, I include a two-minute period when you will be working at your peak of effort and heart rate. For special events we cheerleaders would perform our longest and most intense routines at halftime, and so will you. These workouts are designed to gradually bring you to that peak of effort at halftime and then bring you through a gradual descent—all the way through to your cooldown. Those two minutes are likely to be the toughest for you, but you'll know that, just like when you reach the top of a hill on a hike or a bike ride, the rest is all downhill from there!

Supplies

Not only will you have to devote no more than thirty minutes to your exercise, you don't need any fancy gadgets or elaborate machines. For some of these exercises, I ask that you use free weights. What you will need are two pairs of dumbbells—one pair of lighter weights (one to three pounds) and one heavier (five to eight pounds). You can find these at just about any sporting goods store and they are a worthwhile investment of just a couple dollars. In the exercise descriptions, I will specify whether to use the lighter or the heavier weights. You also must self-monitor.

If you were to do fifteen repetitions with five-pound weights and not feel any sort of fatigue, you must increase your weights. You should start to tire on the last couple reps.

As is true with any exercise, proper breathing technique is important. You should always exhale on the effort. Don't hold your breath when lifting the weight and then exhale when you lower it. Your muscles need the oxygen to do the work you're asking of them. Keep the oxygen-carrying blood pumping to your muscles by exhaling on the effort.

Also, when lifting the weights, don't "throw" them. By that I mean you should raise and lower the weights with slow, controlled movements. Don't let the momentum of the movement carry the weight for you. Challenge the muscle by moving slowly!

Week 1 (Monday, Wednesday, Friday)

Pointers

As with all stretches, avoid quick bouncing movements. Work toward smooth, flowing movements. Concentrate on your breathing and exhale on the stretch and hold your abs in to help you stay balanced on your one leg.

Doing twelve repetitions of the Step Close, Step Open, Plank Walk, and Squat and Counterbalance amounts to about one minute each.

Step Close (12 repetitions)

Target: Front and back of legs (quadriceps and hamstrings)
Start: Stand with feet approximately shoulder-width apart and weight evenly distributed.
Motion: Take one small step forward with the left leg. Raise the right leg up to waist height. Grasp the right leg with both hands interlocking around your knee. Pull your knee in toward your chest. Hold for five seconds, then release. Take three steps and repeat with left leg raised. That is one repetition.

Step close.

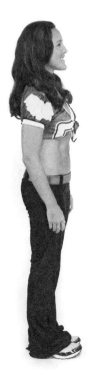
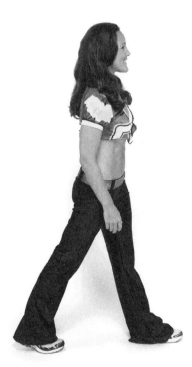
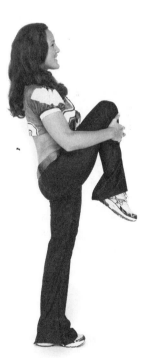

Step Open (12 repetitions)

Target: Front of legs, hips

Start: Stand with feet approximately shoulder-width apart and weight evenly distributed.

Motion: Take one small step forward with the left leg. With your heel leading, raise the right leg up and behind you. Grasp your ankle or top of your foot with the right hand. Gently pull the foot up toward your butt. When you feel a gentle stretch, hold for five seconds and then lower foot. Take three steps and repeat with left leg.

Step open.

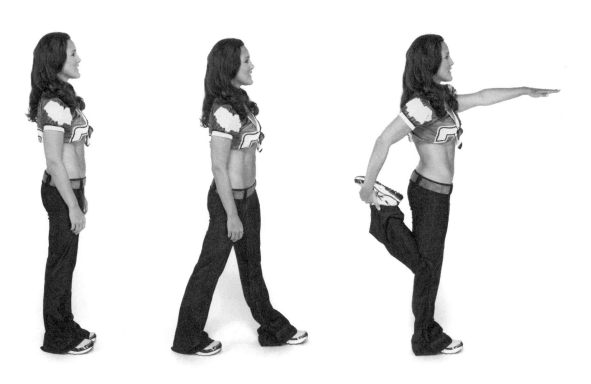

Plank Walk (12 repetitions)

Target: Arms, shoulders, back, core (abs, pelvic floor, hips, and back)

Start: Stand with feet approximately shoulder-width apart and weight evenly distributed.

Motion: From standing position, raise your hands over your head. Exhale and slowly bend at the waist until you are able to place your fingertips on the ground about twelve to eighteen inches in front of your feet, and you can support your weight. Once you've balanced yourself on all fours, slowly walk your hands forward one at a time until your back is nearly parallel to the floor in push-up position. Hold for five seconds and walk hands backward toward your feet. Raise yourself up slowly to the upright position. For this raising motion, imagine that you are a rag doll or a puppet whose strings are slowly being pulled upright.

Plank walk.

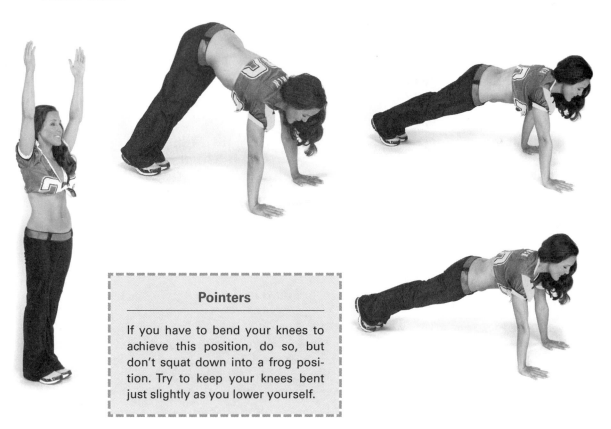

Pointers

If you have to bend your knees to achieve this position, do so, but don't squat down into a frog position. Try to keep your knees bent just slightly as you lower yourself.

Squat and Counterbalance (12 repetitions)

Target: Front of leg, back of leg, shoulders, core (abs, pelvic floor, hips, and back)

Start: Stand with feet approximately shoulder-width apart and weight evenly distributed.

Motion: On the exhale, simultaneously drop your butt and lower yourself into a squatting position until your thighs are parallel to the ground and raise your arms straight out in front of you. Keep your arms in front of you and hold for a five-count and then on the exhale gradually return to the starting position.

Squat and counterbalance.

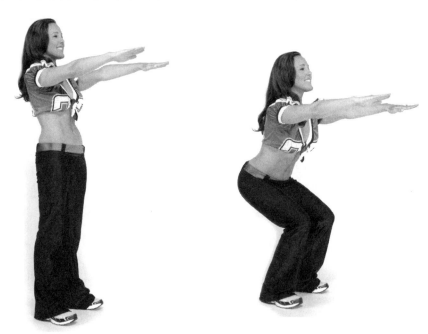

Pointers

Be sure to keep your chin raised and your eyes level throughout the exercise. Use your core muscles to help you lower and raise yourself in control. Going past parallel when squatting is not good on the knees, so stay parallel! To get used to how low to go, you can either do these in front of a mirror or have someone hold his or her hand at the back of your knees so that you just lightly touch it.

BLOCK 1

Zone 1: Transverse Crunch

Target: Core (abs, pelvic floor, hips, and back)

Start: Lie on your back with your knees bent and heels close to your body. Hands are behind the head, with the elbows bent.

Motion: Keeping your lower back on the ground, raise your chest and shoulders toward your knees. At the same time, curl your pelvis toward your rib cage. Lower your back down, but not to the point of relaxation.

Transverse crunch.

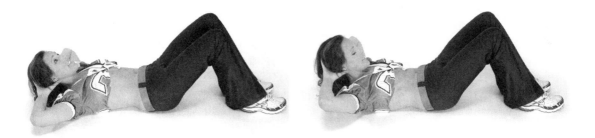

Pointers

Place a hand on your belly to make sure you use your transverse abdominis (the deep abdominal wall). If your belly rises as you perform the exercise, you must readjust and pull your navel down toward your spine. Ideally, your stomach should stay flat as you perform a transverse crunch.

Zone 2: Relevé and Extend

Target: Back of arms, shoulders, calves, upper back

Start: You will need one of your heavier (five- or eight-pound) free weights for this exercise. Stand with feet shoulder-width apart. Holding a free weight with both hands, extend arms over the head, so they are parallel with the ears.

Motion: Keeping your arms next to the ears, bend your elbows, so arms create a 90-degree angle. Then extend arms back up and lift the heels off the ground.

Relevé and extend.

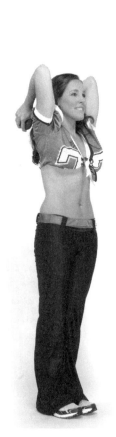 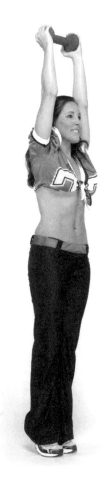

> **Pointers**
>
> Keep your upper arms parallel to your ears and think of your elbows as a locked hinge—they don't move.

Zone 3: Yardline Hop

Target: Cardiovascular exercise

Start: Stand with your feet shoulder-width apart.

Motion: Raise your left leg off the floor with your foot pointed down and slightly behind you. Balancing on one leg, hop two to three times to the left. Lower your left leg, raise your right, and then hop back to the starting point. Continue to alternate legs. Do not rest in between hops. You should continually be in motion.

Yardline hop.

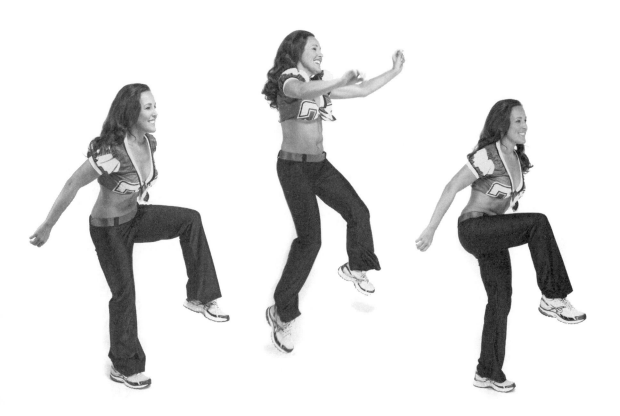

Zone 1: Plié to Passé

Target: Back of legs, butt, inner thighs, outer thighs, front of legs, core (abs, pelvic floor, hips, and back)

Start: Feet are in 1st position, which is heels together, toes turned out, legs squeezed together, butt tight, abs in, shoulders away from the ears.

Motion: Perform a mini plié by bending the knees. Immediately straighten your left leg and bring your right foot toward your knee, with the knee turned out in passé. Perform twenty on each side.

Plié to passé.

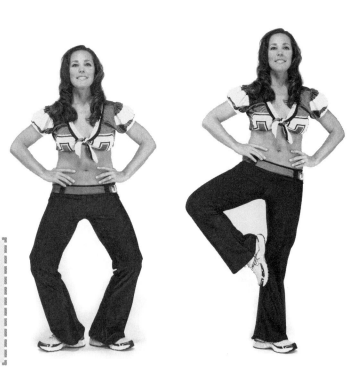

> **Pointers**
>
> You will make the letter P when in passé. Don't forget to keep your abs in. You can say the word "hut" to pull them in.

Zone 2: Lateral Pulldown and Plié

Target: Outer thighs, inner thighs, front of legs, back of legs, butt, back (bra area)

Start: You will need your heavier free weights for this exercise. Stand with legs in a wide stance, toes pointed out. Extend arms above the head, holding the free weights.

Motion: Bend knees and hips. Try to go down so your hips are even with your knees. At the same time, bend elbows and pull down toward the middle of your back. Extend back to the starting position. Keep a neutral spine throughout.

Lateral pulldown and plié.

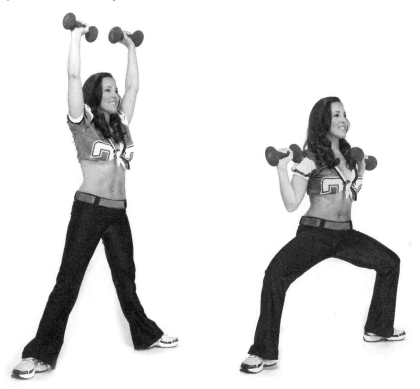

Pointers

Keep your weight in your heels. Do not let knees go past the toes when bending down.

    Beginner modification: Use one arm at a time.

Zone 3: Stair Climb

Target: Cardiovascular exercise

Start: With your feet shoulder-width or less apart, stand in front of a stair.

Motion: Step up with your right leg onto the first stair and then bring the left leg onto the stair. Step back to the ground with your left leg and then your right.

Stair climb.

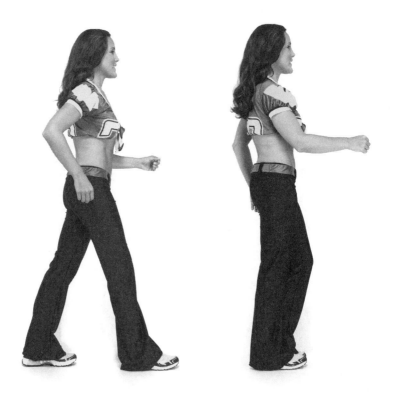

Pointers

Do not rest in between steps. Be sure to alternate the leg you lead with. For a more intense workout you can use a sturdy box or anything else you can safely stand on that is higher than a stair.

Zone 1: Heel Jacks

Target: Legs, hips, butt, heart (cardiovascular exercise)

Start: Stand with your feet together and arms at your sides.

Motion: Keeping your foot lightly in contact with the ground, extend one heel straight out to the side while simultaneously raising your arms to the sides and level with your shoulders. Return to start position. Switch legs and repeat. Add a hop when extending the leg to increase heart rate slightly.

Heel jacks.

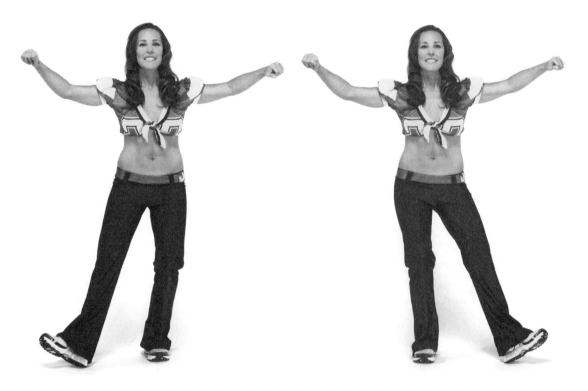

Zone 2: Plié and Handoff

Target: Outer thighs, inner thighs, front of legs, back of legs, butt, core (abs, pelvic floor, hips, and back), shoulders, upper back

Start: Stand with your legs in a greater than shoulder-width stance with toes pointed out. Hold one of your heavier weights in both hands. Bend your knees and hips. Try to lower yourself so that your hips are even with your knees. Extend your arms in front of your body at shoulder height. Keep your back straight and your navel pulled in. Hold your weight in both hands in front of you.

Motion: Keeping your lower body motionless, rotate your torso from side to side, with your arms leading the twist. Do not release the plié until you have completed all repetitions.

Plié and handoff.

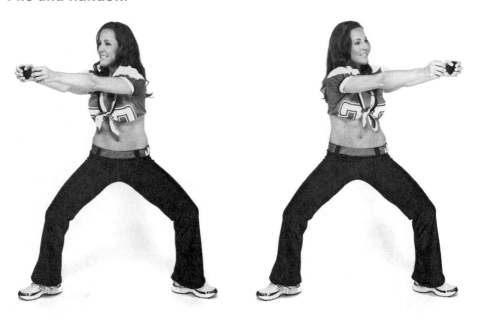

Pointers

Plant feet and hips firmly and move from the waist.

Beginner modification: Use your lighter weight.

Zone 3: Ski

Target: Cardiovascular exercise

Start: Stand with your feet shoulder-width apart. Place your hands on your hips.

Motion: Hop and bring your right foot in front of you. Hop and return to the starting position. Hop with the left foot moving forward. Do not rest in between hops.

Ski.

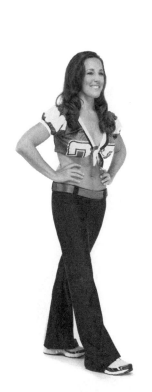 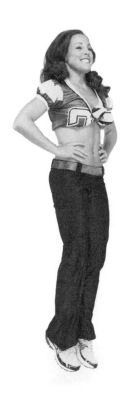 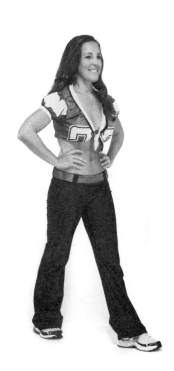

HALFTIME BREAK: KICK SEQUENCE

Perform a kick sequence for two minutes by placing your hands on your hips with your elbows bent. Hop with your feet together. Then lift your right knee, hop with your feet together, then lift with your left knee, hop with feet together, lift right leg to kick waist height, hop with feet together, lift left leg to kick waist height. Exhale every time you lift a leg!

Halftime kick sequence.

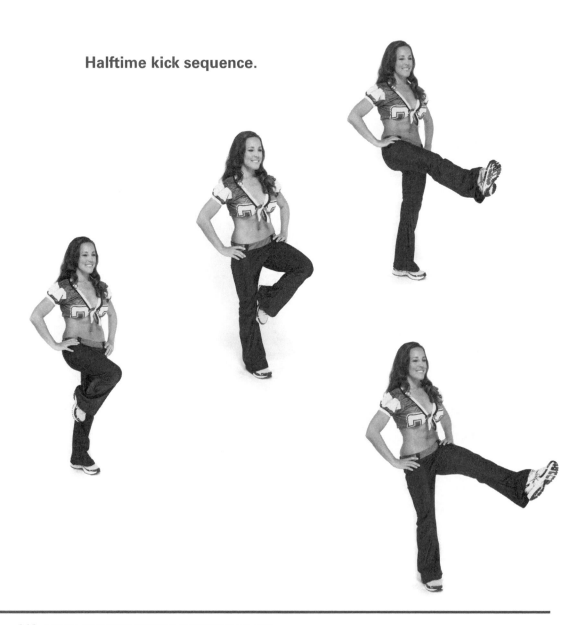

Zone 1: Biceps Curl with Core Balance

Target: Front of arms, core (abs, pelvic floor, hips, back), upper back

Start: You need your heavier free weights for this exercise. Stand with your feet a few inches apart and a free weight in each hand. Keep your upper arms and elbows gently pressed against your body for the duration of the exercise and one knee stays lifted.

Motion: With your palms facing out, exhale and bring the weights toward your shoulders. Keep a neutral (straight) spine, by pulling your abs toward your spine. Inhale as you lower the weights. Repeat ten times, exhaling each time you lift the weights and inhaling as you lower them. Lift your left leg and do ten more curls. Then repeat ten more with right leg raised. Try not to let your elbows leave your sides and do not bend the wrists.

Biceps curl with core balance.

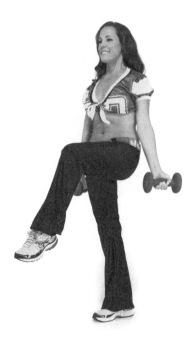 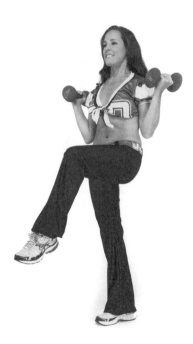

Zone 2: Curtsy Core Isolation

Target: Inner thighs, outer thighs, butt, core (abs, pelvic floor, hips, and back), shoulders

Start: Stand with your feet shoulder-width apart. Extend your arms in front of your body at shoulder height. Shift your weight onto your right leg.

Motion: Extend your left leg one or two feet behind you, diagonally, with your heel lifted. Bend your knees to a 90-degree angle. Return to starting position and alternate legs.

Curtsy core isolation.

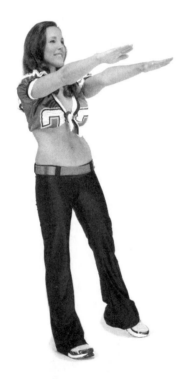
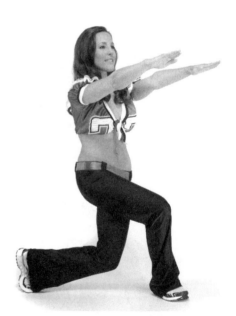

Pointers

Bend both knees and keep your front heel on the ground. Do not let your knees go forward past the toes when bending down.

Zone 3: Cross-Jacks

Target: Cardiovascular exercise

Start: Begin with your feet together.

Motion: Do a traditional jumping jack, but cross your feet one in front of the other when you come back to the center. Alternate which foot you cross in front of the other and do not rest between jumps.

Cross-jacks.

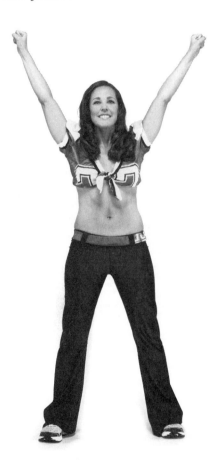
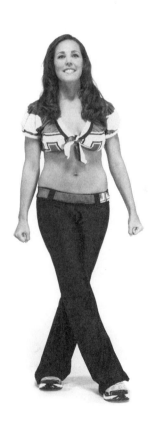

Zone 1: Chest Press and Crunch

Target: Chest, core (abs, pelvic floor, hips, and back), shoulders

Start: You will need your heavier free weights for this exercise. Lie on your back with your knees bent and heels close to your butt. Place arms palms-down on the floor at a 90-degree angle to your body, holding a free weight in each hand. Elbows should be even with the shoulders and your neck should not be scrunched.

Motion: Crunch up, simultaneously lifting your hands until they are directly above your elbows. Squeeze your chest muscles as you raise your upper body and cross your arms at the elbows. Extend and release.

Chest press and crunch.

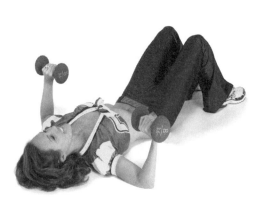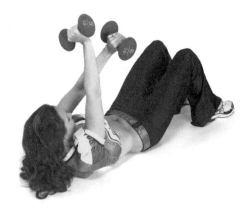

Pointers

Use your transverse abs by pulling the belly in and down. Emphasize the chest squeeze.

Zone 2: Goalpost Squat

Target: Front of legs, back of legs, butt, shoulders, back of arms, core (abs, pelvic floor, hips, and back)

Start: You will need your heavier free weights for this exercise. Stand with feet shoulder-width apart (or slightly more). Extend your arms above your head, holding a free weight in each hand.

Motion: Bend at the hips slightly, then lower yourself so that your knees are at a 90-degree angle. Simultaneously bring arms down: first bending elbows and holding weights up at shoulder height, then lowering the weights straight down at your sides. Raise yourself to the standing position, while pressing your arms up above your head.

Goalpost squat.

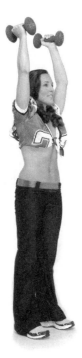
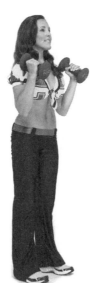
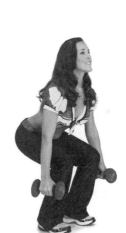

Pointers

Most of your weight should be in your heels, almost lifting the toes. Do not let knees go forward past the toes when bending down. Keep your abs pulled in with your navel toward your spine. Focus on using your shoulder muscles to lift the weight above your head.

Zone 3: Football Shuffle

Target: Cardiovascular exercise
Start: Stand with your feet comfortably spread.
Motion: Run in place, bringing your knees up gradually higher.

Football shuffle.

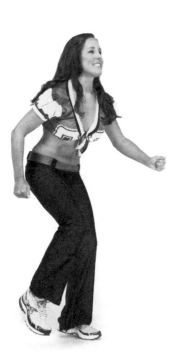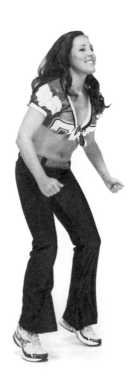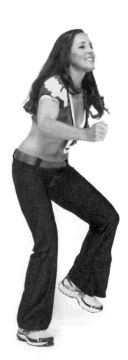

Pointers

While lifting your knees up as high as you can does increase the intensity of the workout, you can also increase your tempo (what runners call turnover) to achieve the same result. In other words, the more times you bring your feet up and down, the more intense the exercise.

BLOCK 6

Zone 1: Inner-Thigh Adductions

Target: Inner thighs, core (abs, pelvic floor, hips, and back)

Start: Lie on your back. Place your arms above your head in a U shape. Pull your navel toward your spine, so your lower back stays on the ground. Lift both legs above the hips, so that the hips are slightly flexed. Pull your toes toward your shins, so that your feet are flexed, too.

Motion: Starting at center, open your legs out to the sides and then bring them back together.

Inner-thigh adductions.

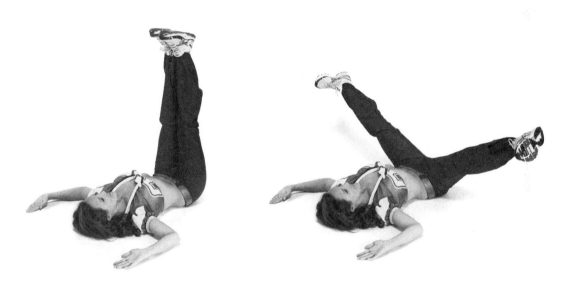

Pointers

Use your transverse abs by pulling the belly in and down.

Zone 2: Woodchop to Squat

Target: Front of legs, back of legs, butt, shoulders, back of arms, core (abs, pelvic floor, hips, and back), upper back

Start: You will need one of your heavier free weights for this exercise. Stand with feet hip-width apart. Holding one weight with both hands, extend arms up and across the body in a diagonal line.

Motion: Keeping arms straight, pull them down and across the body. Using your core to pull down the arms, begin to squat. (Bend the hips slightly, then bend the knees to create a 90-degree angle.) Arms follow the diagonal back up to standing. Be sure to switch arms and do the other side after twenty reps.

Woodchop to squat.

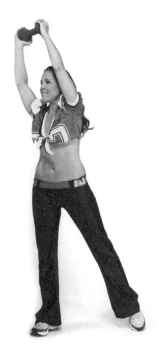
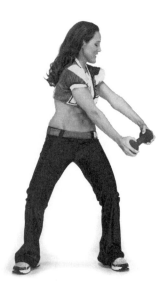

Pointers

Use your core for this motion and keep your abs pulled in. Most of your weight should be in your heels, almost lifting the toes. Do not let knees go past the toes when bending down.

Zone 3: Bounder

Target: Cardiovascular exercise

Start: Stand with your legs shoulder-width apart with your arms hanging at your sides.

Motion: Lift one knee at a time while raising your opposite arm above your head. Bring your foot back to the floor, lowering your arm as you do so.

Bounder.

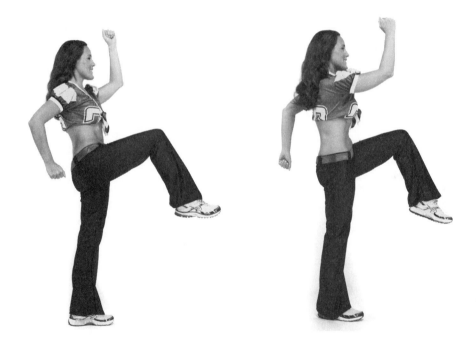

Pointers

Each time you lift a knee, raise your opposite arm, and each time you lower the knee, lower the arm. Do not rest in between.

AB 5 (SEE PAGE 165)

YOGA COOLDOWN (SEE PAGE 250)

Notice how in the fat-burning zone, I had you move through each of the three effort/heart rate zones. This is interval training at its best and most efficient. Not only will this help your mind stay active and alert, but it will efficiently help you to burn calories generally and fat calories specifically.

Week 2 (Monday, Wednesday, Friday)

Do: Warm-up, Block 2, Block 3, Block 4, Halftime, Block 5, Block 6, Ab 5,
   Yoga Cooldown
Don't do: Block 1
Add: Block 7

Zone 1: Modified Boomerang

Target: core (abs, pelvic floor, hips, and back), upper back, shoulders

Start: Get in the prone position. Place your elbows on the ground directly under your shoulders with your legs bent.

Motion: Raise yourself so that your body is supported by your knees and elbows. Pull your navel in so you maintain a straight line from the top of the head to the toes. Hold this position. Rotate and drop one hip toward the ground, then the other. Keep your hips close to the ground as you rotate.

Modified boomerang.

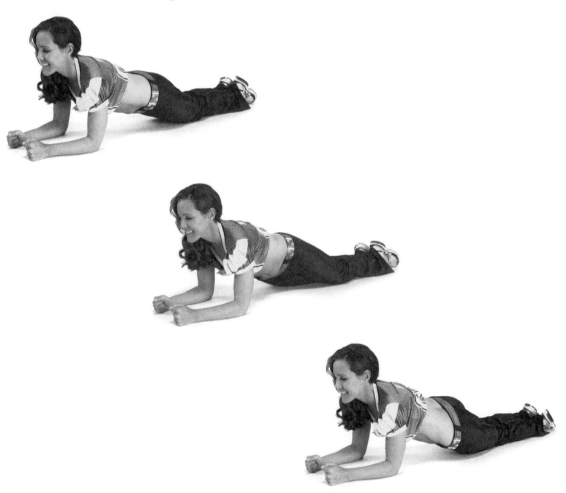

Zone 2: Football Push-up

Target: Chest, core (abs, pelvic floor, hips, and back), shoulders, front of arms, back of arms, upper back

Start: Lie on the floor facedown, using your arms to hold yourself up (palms placed wider than shoulder-width flat on the floor). Keep your head neutral. Your arms and back are supporting you, your knees are on the ground, and your core is tight.

Motion: Bend elbows away from the body, lowering yourself to the ground. Straighten elbows. Walk both hands about a foot to one side. Repeat push-up, then walk hands to starting position. Alternate sides.

Football push-up.

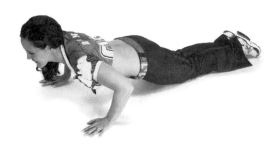

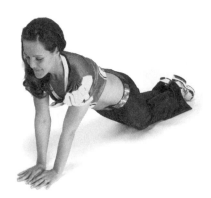

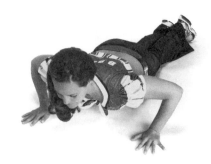

Pointers

Wider arms target more chest muscles. Try to keep your shoulders directly over your wrists.

Zone 3: Wide Run

Target: Cardiovascular exercise

Starting Position: Stand with your feet a little wider apart than your shoulders. Bend at the waist slightly but keep your chin in place. Arms should be hanging at your sides.

Motion: Begin running in place, lifting your feet six to twelve inches off the floor. Form a soft fist with each hand and bring them to chest level. The object here is speed. Get your feet moving as fast as possible. You will not be raising your knees very high.

Wide run.

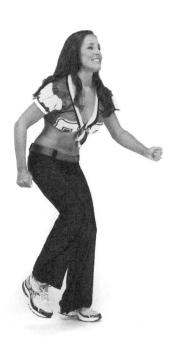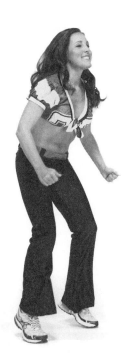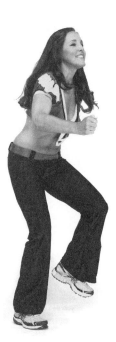

Do: Warm-up, Block 3, Block 4, Block 5, Halftime, Block 6, Block 7, Ab 5, Yoga Cooldown

Don't do: Block 1, Block 2

Add: Block 8

BLOCK 8

Zone 1: Bridge Knee Abduction

Target: Outer thighs, back of legs, butt, inner thighs

Start: Lie on your back with your knees bent and heels twelve to eighteen inches from your butt. Arms should be by your sides, palms facedown.

Motion: Squeeze your knees together and exhale while raising your pelvis about twelve inches off the ground. Slowly lower your body and open your knees to the sides. Keep your feet on the ground. Release until your knees are a few inches above the ground, and then bring your knees back together. Squeeze the knees and butt in the starting position.

Bridge knee abduction.

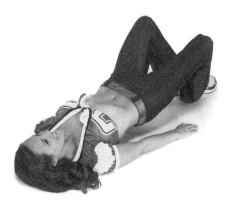 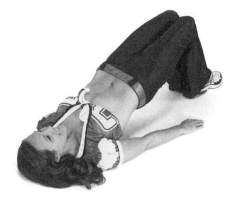

Zone 2: Triceps Dip

Target: Back of arms, upper back, shoulders, chest

Start: Sit on the floor, with your palms flat on the ground and your elbows bent at a 90-degree angle.

Motion: With feet and hands on the ground, push your torso up with your arms. Raise and lower the torso, by bending and straightening the arms.

Triceps dip.

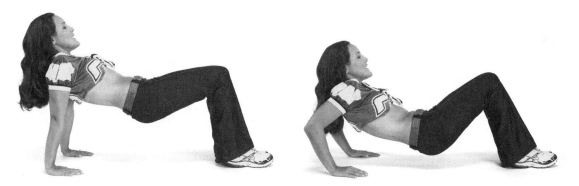

Pointers

Try to bend elbows to 90 degrees and keep the majority of your weight on your arms.

Beginner modification: Place your hands on a stair or step.

Advanced modification: Keep your legs straight in front of you instead of bent.

Zone 3: Plyometric Tuck Jump

Target: Cardiovascular exercise

Start: Stand with your feet six to twelve inches apart. Place your hands on your hips.

Motion: Bend slightly at the knees and then jump straight up, bringing your knees toward your chest.

Plyometric tuck jump.

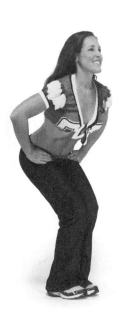 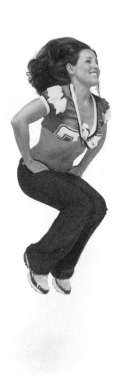

Pointers

Keep your chin up and focus on a point across the room from you. Do not pause between jumps.

   Beginner modification: Bring one knee up at a time while raising your arms over your head.

AB 5 (SERIES OF FIVE EXERCISES)

Target: Core (abs, pelvic floor, hips, and back)

Start: Lying on your back, except for the back hyperextension, which you start by lying facedown.

Motion: See descriptions below.

Pointers

Keep your abs pulled in and down, so the lower back is anchored through all of these exercises. This is very important to make sure you are targeting the right muscles and to protect the lower back. Always breathe out on the exertion (raising yourself up) and breathe in on the rest (lowering yourself). Aim for twenty repetitions.

Elbow Tap

Sit on your "sitz" bones with your knees and hips flexed. Round your back and look at your navel. Extend both hands in front of you and pull back one elbow at a time so that it makes light contact with the floor. Hold your abs firm, and try to keep your legs and torso as still as possible.

Elbow tap (Ab 5).

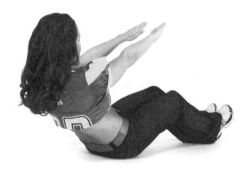

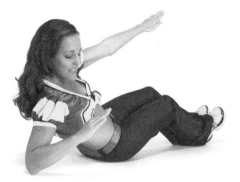

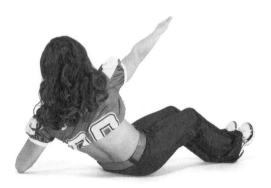

Scissor

Lie on your back and place your hands under your butt, palms down. While keeping your lower back on the floor, raise both your feet in the air above your hips with your legs straight. Lower one leg 45 degrees and bring back to center. Switch legs.

Scissor (Ab 5).

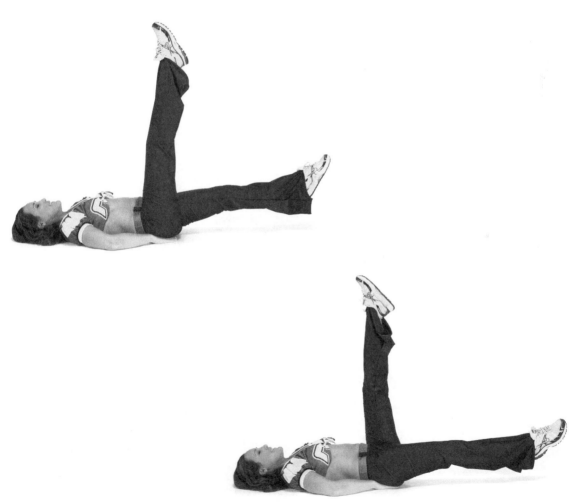

Scissor with Upper Body Twist

Lie on your back. While keeping your lower back on the floor, raise both of your feet in the air above your hips with your legs straight. Lower your right leg 45 degrees and twist your upper body to the left. Come back to center. Alternate legs. Lower your left leg 45 degrees and twist your upper body to the right. Interlock your hands behind your head and keep your elbows behind your ears while you twist.

Scissor with upper body twist (Ab 5).

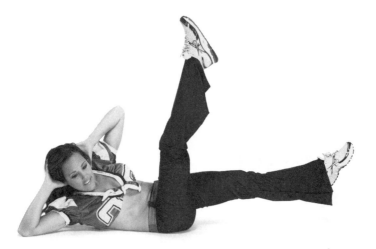

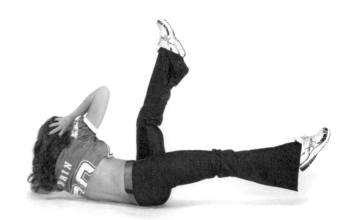

Bicycle

Lie on your back. Place your hands behind your head and keep your elbows back. Bring your right knee toward your chest and twist and raise your left shoulder up and toward your knee. Keep the left leg straight and held off the ground at a height according to your strength. The higher you hold the straight leg off the ground, the easier the exercise will be; the lower you raise that leg, the more difficult it will be. Alternate sides to create a motion like you are riding a bike.

Bicycle (Ab 5).

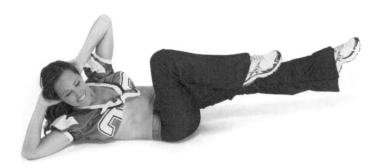

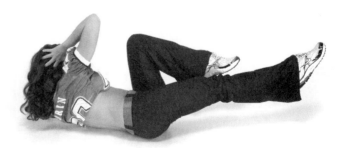

Back Hyperextension

Lie facedown with your arms extended forward, your elbows by your ears, and your feet together. Lift your upper body and lower body simultaneously. Lower yourself back to the starting position.

Back hyperextension (Ab 5).

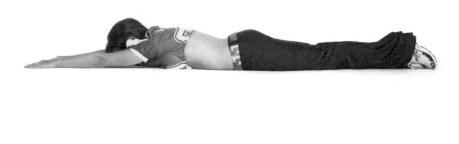

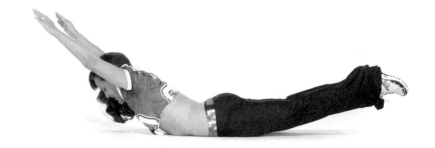

For each of the three weeks in Phase 1, you can choose whatever cardio exercise you prefer to do on the days I've designated the Cardio Zone days. On Tuesdays and Thursdays, the idea is to get your heart rate up with some sustained cardiovascular activity. After a brief warm-up, you should stay in Zone 2, working at a perceived exertion of 5 to 7 or a heart rate of 70–80 percent of your target heart rate. Unlike with the fat-burning zone, you won't really be doing intervals when you are going into and out of that highest effort, Zone 3. As you will see, though, you will alternate somewhat in terms of walking versus jogging, etc. Varying your *pace* and not your *intensity level* is what you're after here.

Following are several options for your cardio workouts.

Walk, Jog, or Run Outside: 30 minutes

Follow one of these interval patterns:

Walking: Walk four minutes, jog one minute. Repeat six times.
Jogging/running: Walk three minutes to warm up. Then jog three minutes, run one minute; repeat seven times.

If at all possible, please avoid running and jogging on concrete. It is an incredibly hard surface, and your feet and joints will pay the price. A composition running track is soft, and grass is softer, but if those aren't available to you, asphalt pavement is better than a concrete sidewalk.

Treadmill: 30 minutes total

You will alternate doing two different levels of intensity (speed) and incline:

Level 1—First two minutes, easy walking at an incline of 1 and speed of one to three miles per hour.
Level 2—Second two minutes, jog or briskly walk at an incline of 5 and a speed of four to five miles per hour.

Do seven sets alternating the level 1 and level 2 treadmill work, ending with a two-minute cooldown.

Please note: Because most treadmill work is done indoors and you don't have wind or inclines to make the work easier or harder, you should never walk or run on the treadmill without the incline being set to *at least* 1. When the treadmill isn't raised, it simulates going downhill. Don't cheat yourself by going downhill or by holding on to the rails.

Elliptical Trainer: 30 minutes

Warm-up: Three easy minutes

Workout: Spend three minutes at a steady pace, then increase your pace for two minutes—go fast. Repeat until thirty minutes is reached. Increase your resistance for more of a challenge. Remember, you're putting in the time, so put in the effort as well!

I recommend the elliptical trainer instead of the treadmill or running/jogging outdoors for people who have problems with either their hips, knees, ankles, or feet. The elliptical trainer eliminates some of the pounding associated with running and jogging. You get more of a calorie burn while running, which is why if you use the elliptical trainer I have you working out in Zone 3 and not in Zone 2, but it can be hard on the joints.

CARDIO CHEATERS NEVER WIN AND CARDIO WINNERS NEVER CHEAT

Of course, when we're kids we heard a different version of this mantra all the time. As adults we don't always consciously cheat, but we sometimes slip up and do things we shouldn't. Well, my variation on this little pearl of wisdom applies in two very specific situations. When running on a treadmill or using an elliptical trainer, or even a stairclimber, if you rest any part of your weight on the hand rails, you are cheating yourself! (Incidentally, I don't advise you to use a stair climber unless nothing else is available. Why? Because it is so easy to cheat on one of these machines and stair climbing can really be bad on hips, knees, and ankles.)

When you support yourself or any part of your weight on the machine itself, you are not working as hard as you could be (and should be) because your legs aren't moving your full weight. Studies have shown that leaning on the machine can make your exercise as much as 20 to 50 percent less efficient!

Again, let your own level of pain be your guide. If you are having difficultly breathing while running, or if you get a stitch in your side, that's discomfort.

If you feel a sharp and persistent pain in one of your joints, that's pain with a capital P. I don't want you to be in pain, but you should get used to working through some discomfort.

Stationary Cycle: 30 Minutes

This is another easy piece of equipment to start out on without the joint impact of running outdoors or the treadmill. A few things to keep in mind when working out on the stationary cycle: Adjust the seat to your body. When you sit on the cycle's seat with your foot on the pedal in its lowest position, there should only be a slight bend in your knee, approximately 25–35 degrees. Watch your form. Pay close attention to your upper body position: Don't slouch over the handlebars! Keep your upper body high, with your shoulders relaxed and your head up. Don't be afraid to stand and pedal. If you're really getting into your ride and want to vary the intensity, crank up the resistance and pedal while standing out of your seat. It adds some variety and helps prevent a sore butt from sitting too long.

Warm-up: For five minutes, pedal slowly, without resistance, concentrating on your form and gradually start building speed to a level that puts you into your Zone 2 heart rate.

Workout: For twenty minutes, vary your speed and resistance but maintain your Zone 2 heart rate throughout this period.

Cooldown: Over five minutes, gradually slow your pedaling speed and reduce resistance. Don't stop abruptly; use this time to let your body cool off and get your heart rate down. As your heart rate begins to decrease, let go of the handlebars, sit upright, and loosen up your upper body. Try doing neck and shoulder rolls, stretch your torso by reaching up to the ceiling with your hands, and cross your arms in front and give yourself a hug while you stretch out your upper back.

Kickboxing or Aerobics Class

You also can take a kickboxing or aerobics class on Cardio Zone days.

THE BUDDY SYSTEM

Working out with someone else or in a class is a great way to stay motivated. The problem with working out with a buddy or in a group is always scheduling. One thing you can do to create a gymlike buddy atmosphere is to listen to music while you exercise. Since I love to dance so much, music is a *huge* part of my life and my workouts. Here's a recent iPod playlist that's a mix of all-time faves and recent tunes to get my heart pumping and my fat-burning engine running:

Theme from the movie *Rocky*
O.A.R.: "That Was a Crazy Game of Poker" and "Love and Memories"
Fleetwood Mac: "Everywhere"
Danity Kane: "Show Stopper"
Murphy Lee, Nelly, and P. Diddy: "Shake Ya Tailfeather"
The Samples: "Did You Ever Look So Nice"
Coldplay: "Viva la Vida"
Nelly: "Country Grammar" and "Over and Over"
Murphy Lee: "Wat Da Hook Gon Be" and "Luv Me Baby"
Sean Paul: "Get Busy"
Rihanna: "Pon de Replay"
Salt 'N' Pepa: "Push It"
Tina Turner: "Proud Mary"
Kelis: "Milkshake"
Nelly Furtado: "Maneater"
Jay-Z: "Big Pimpin'"
Barry White: "Can't Get Enough of Your Love, Babe"
Louis Armstrong: "What a Wonderful World"

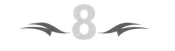

THE ULTIMATE SIX-WEEK FITNESS PLAN

Phase 2—

The "Get into Your Fat-Burning Zone" Workout

Congratulations! You did it! You got through the first twenty-one days of the Ultimate Six-Week Fitness Plan! I told you before that most people abandon their exercise and nutrition plans within the first three weeks. Once they get beyond that point, they tend to stick with them for the long term. You should be really proud of yourself for making it this far. You've put up with some tender muscles, modified your eating habits, been faithful to keeping your food journal, and, I hope, seen the results you were hoping for—weight loss, toning, improved energy, and endurance.

By now, I hope that you look forward to your workouts and have also realized some of the side benefits of exercising—reduced stress and better rest. Also, at this stage engaging your transverse abdominis muscles, breathing from your diaphragm, exhaling on the effort, and staying balanced and in control with your movements have become second nature to you.

If you're not losing the weight you want, it's time to get serious about your food journal! And count those calories!

Since variety, as the saying goes, is the spice of life, I have a method behind my madness in Phase 2 of our six-week fitness plan. New routines with different exercises and different emphases are important to keep your mind engaged and help you avoid ruts. More important, there are some physical reasons why we have to raise your game to another level.

As I have said before, as you work your way through this program, you will be getting more fit, your resting heart rate will likely have improved, and it will take a little more effort to get into your Zone 2 and Zone 3 heart rate. You don't want to plateau and not realize the same benefits as you did when you first started. For that reason, we're going to mix things up a bit, with the exception of your warm-up exercises. For Phase 2, you will continue to use Step Close, Step Open, Plank Walk, and Squat and Counterbalance in weeks 4 through 6.

The good news is that you will still only need to devote a half hour a day to your exercise routine, just as you did before. This means that you'll be picking up the intensity a bit, but not increasing the total amount of time you have to devote to exercise. That's the great thing about interval training. You simply adjust the time you spend in the different zones without extending the total time you exercise. In other words, you can achieve greater benefits in the same amount of time!

After you review this schedule, I'll talk to you a bit more about nutrition for Phase 2.

Week 4 (Monday, Wednesday, Friday)

WARM-UP

Doing twelve repetitions of the Step Close, Step Open, Plank Walk, and Squat and Counterbalance amounts to about one minute each.

Step Close (12 repetitions)

Target: Front and back of legs (quadriceps and hamstrings)

Start: Stand with feet approximately shoulder-width apart and weight evenly distributed.

Motion: Take one small step forward with the left leg. Raise the right leg up to waist height. Grasp the right leg with both hands interlocking around your knee. Pull your knee in toward your chest. Hold for five seconds. Take three steps forward and repeat with your left leg raised.

Step close.

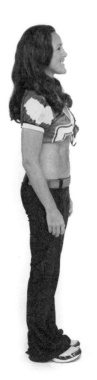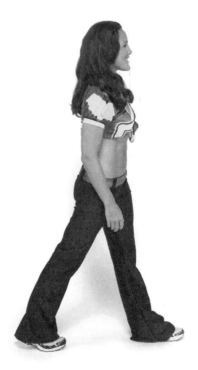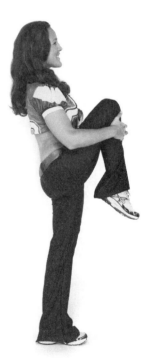

Step Open (12 repetitions)

Target: Front of leg (quadriceps), hips

Start: Stand with feet approximately shoulder-width apart and weight evenly distributed.

Motion: Take one small step forward with the left leg. With your heel leading, raise the right leg up and behind you. Grasp your ankle or top of your foot with the right hand. Gently pull the foot up toward your butt. When you feel a gentle stretch, hold for five seconds and then lower your foot. Take three steps forward and repeat with your left leg.

Step open.

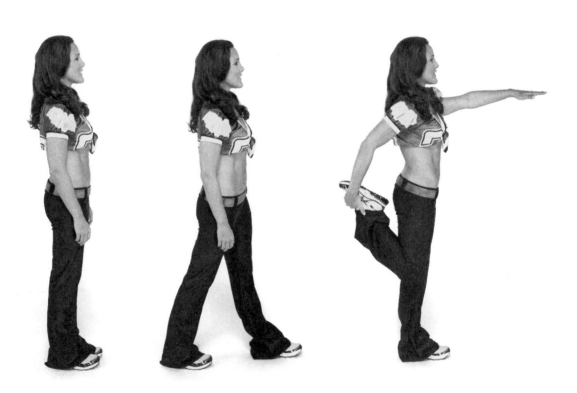

Plank Walk (12 repetitions)

Target: Arms, shoulders, back, core (abs, pelvic floor, hips, and back)

Start: Stand with feet approximately shoulder-width apart and weight evenly distributed.

Motion: From standing position, raise your hands over your head. Exhale and slowly bend at the waist until you are able to place your fingertips on the ground about twelve to eighteen inches in front of your feet, and you can support your weight. Once you've balanced yourself on all fours, slowly walk your hands forward one at a time until your back is nearly parallel to the floor in push-up position. Hold for five seconds and walk hands backward toward your feet. Raise yourself up slowly to the upright position. For this raising motion, imagine that you are a rag doll or a puppet whose strings are slowly being pulled upright.

Plank walk.

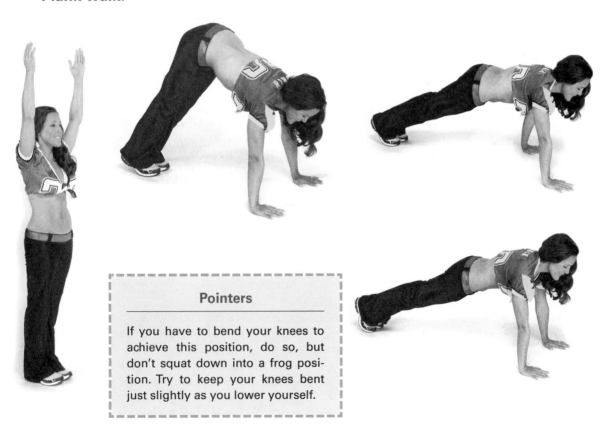

Pointers

If you have to bend your knees to achieve this position, do so, but don't squat down into a frog position. Try to keep your knees bent just slightly as you lower yourself.

Squat and Counterbalance (12 repetitions)

Target: Front of leg, back of leg

Start: Stand with feet approximately shoulder-width apart and weight evenly distributed.

Motion: On the exhale, simultaneously drop your butt and lower yourself into a squatting position until your thighs are parallel to the ground and raise your arms straight out in front of you. Hold for a five-count and then on the exhale gradually return to the starting position, but keep your arms out in front of you.

Squat and counterbalance.

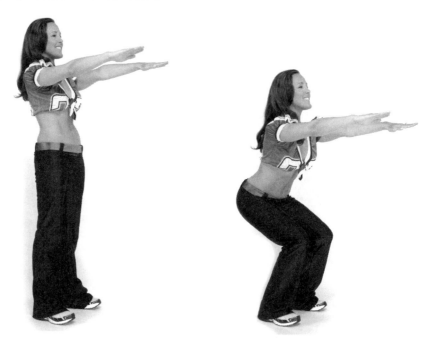

Pointers

Be sure to keep your chin raised and your eyes level throughout the exercise. Use your core muscles to help you lower and raise yourself in control. Going past parallel when squatting is not good on the knees, so stay parallel! To get used to how low to go, you can either do these in front of a mirror or have someone hold his or her hand at the back of your knees so that you just lightly touch it.

BLOCK 9

Zone 1: Chest Fly and Bridge

Target: Chest, back of legs, butt, core (abs, pelvic floor, hips, and back)

Start: You will need your heavier weights. Lie in supine (on back) position with your knees bent and heels twelve to eighteen inches from your butt. Raise your hips off the ground in a bridge. Place your elbows at a 90-degree bend in line with your shoulders. Your palms should face each other.

Motion: Extend your arms and bring your hands together directly above your midline. Squeeze your chest muscles; extend and release arms, maintaining the bridge position.

Chest fly and bridge.

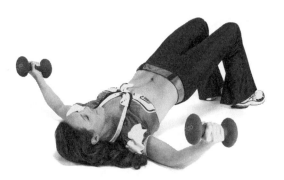 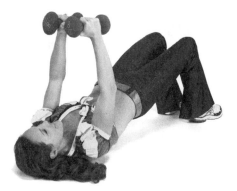

Pointers

Emphasize the chest squeeze. Do not let the hips drop.

Zone 2: Mermaid

Target: Core (abs—especially the obliques—pelvic floor, hips, and back) shoulders, upper back

Start: Lie on your side with your legs straight. Cross one foot over the other and let it lie flat. Place your bottom hand palm down on the ground. Lift your hips so that your body forms a diagonal line. Push out of the floor to keep your head from resting on your shoulder. Try not to roll forward or back.

Motion: From the side plank position, lift your hips straight up and down. Try not to roll forward. Use your obliques (waistline) to lift. Return to side plank position. Be sure to switch sides and do twenty repetitions on the other side.

Mermaid.

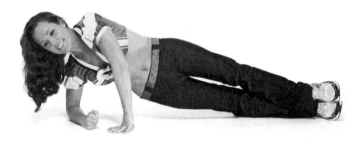

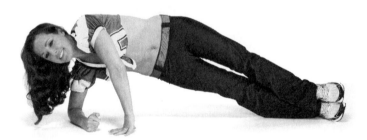

Pointers

Beginner modification: Instead of the plank/push-up position, rest on your knees.

Zone 3: Kick Line

Target: Cardiovascular exercise

Start: Stand with your feet shoulder-width apart and extend your arms out to the sides so they are even with your shoulders.

Motion: Kick your right leg in front of you. Bring your right foot back to the ground and keep your arms even with your shoulders. Switch legs and repeat.

Kick line.

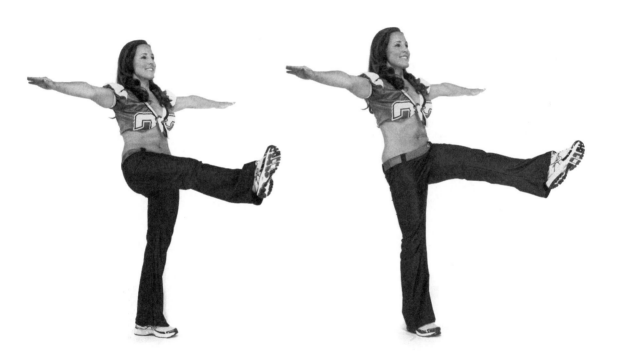

Pointers

This is a very rhythmic dancelike movement. Keep bouncing throughout and don't rest when you bring your foot back down. As soon as that left leg touches the ground, get the other one in the air right away!

Zone 1: Attitude Lifts

Target: Back of legs, butt, inner thighs, outer thighs, front of legs, core (abs, pelvic floor, hips, and back), shoulders

Start: Hinge upper body forward slightly and bring right leg up and behind you. Bend the right leg to 90 degrees and turn out so the inside of your knee faces the ground. Arms are locked out to your sides at shoulder height.

Motion: Keep the right leg in this attitude while pulling the quadriceps (the muscle above your knee) tight on your left leg. Lift the right leg up and down a few inches.

Attitude lifts.

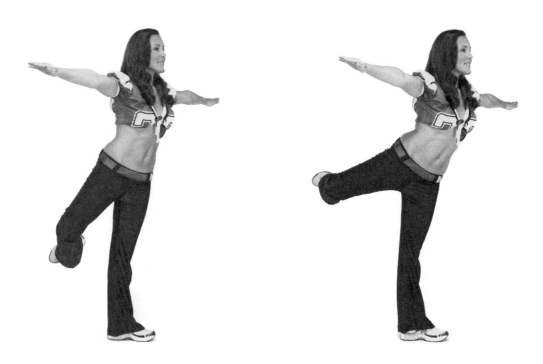

Pointers

Squeeze the hips and butt to keep the attitude position. You will feel your core working—keep your abs in!

Zone 2: Plié and Relevé

Target: Outer thighs, inner thighs, butt, calves, and core (abs, pelvic floor, hips, and back)

Start: You will need one of your heavier weights. Place your feet wider than shoulder-width apart with your toes pointed out. Bend knees and flex hips so that your hips are at the same height as your knees. Holding one end of the weight with each hand, drop your arms so that they are fully extended between your legs.

Motion: Lift your heels and extend your ankles. Return by releasing your heels to the floor.

Plié and relevé.

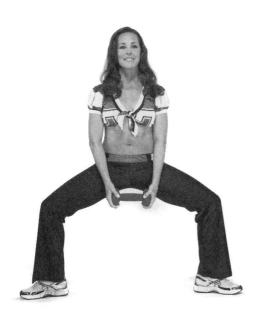 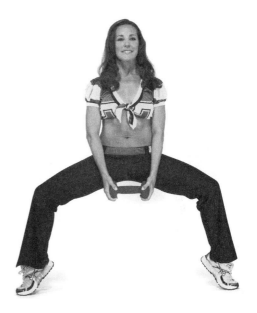

Pointers

Keep your back straight and your navel pulled in.

Zone 3: Squat Thrust

Target: Cardiovascular exercise
Start: Stand with your feet six to twelve inches apart and your hands at your sides.
Motion: Squat down so that your hands are on the floor about twelve inches in front of your feet and shoulder-width apart. Keep your chin up. Kick both legs back into the push-up position. Make sure that your hands are directly beneath your shoulders. Kick your legs forward so that you return to the squatting position. Stand up while bringing your hands directly over your head with your palms facing forward.

Squat thrust.

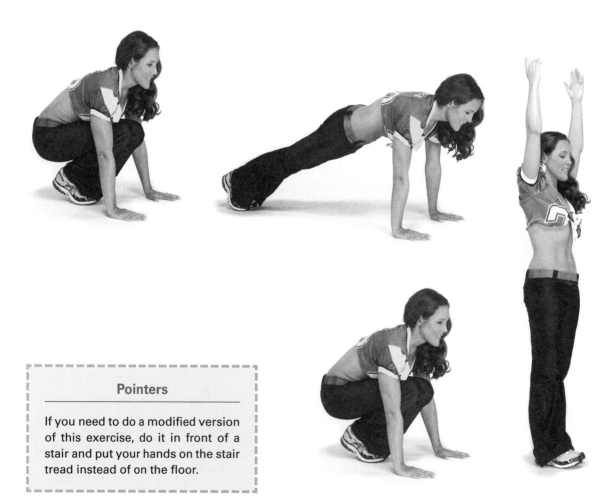

Pointers

If you need to do a modified version of this exercise, do it in front of a stair and put your hands on the stair tread instead of on the floor.

Zone 1: Triceps Kickback in Extended Warrior

Target: Core (abs, pelvic floor, hips, and back), back of arms, upper back, butt, back of legs, back of shoulders

Start: You will need your lighter free weights. Begin by assuming the Extended Warrior position: with your feet shoulder-width apart, extend your right leg behind your body and tilt your torso forward approximately 30 degrees to maintain your balance. Hold weights in both hands. Elevate your bent elbows above your hips with your palms facing forward. Your upper arms should be slightly above your torso. Your arms should form 90-degree angles.

Motion: Fully extend your arms behind you while keeping your elbows at the same height. Hold for one second using the triceps muscle. Release your arms into their 90-degree starting position, but do not lower your leg or change your position. Keep abs in. Do ten repetitions, then switch legs and do ten more.

Triceps kickback in Extended Warrior.

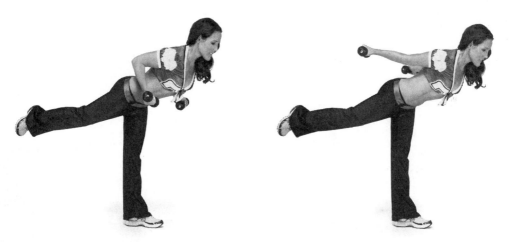

Pointers

The higher you raise your elbows in the starting position, the more intensely you will work your triceps muscles. If this irritates your back, you can do one arm at a time. You can also support your back by placing one hand on your knee and not lifting your leg (but do lean your torso forward).

Zone 2: Reverse Lunge to Biceps Curl

Target: Front of arms, butt, legs

Start: You will need both of your heavier weights. Stand with your feet shoulder-width apart. Keep your elbows close to your body, palms facing forward, with a weight in each hand.

Motion: Step back two to three feet with your left leg. Bend both your knees to 90 degrees and slightly flex hips. Simultaneously bend your elbows and curl your palms toward the shoulders. Contract your biceps muscles and extend your arms while you return your legs to the starting position. Switch lead legs and do twenty repetitions on the other side, but this time without the biceps curls.

Reverse lunge to biceps curl.

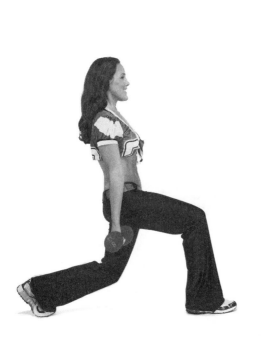
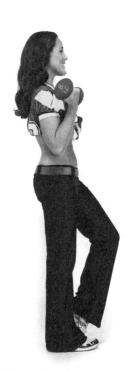

Pointers

Keep a majority of your weight on the front foot and keep your knee directly over your heel. While curling the weights, keep your elbows still and tucked in toward your body.

Zone 3: Hurdler

Target: Cardiovascular exercise

Start: Stand with your feet comfortably apart and your hands at your sides.

Motion: Squat down with your hands on the floor just in front of your feet. Raise your butt into the air and walk your hands slightly forward until you are in a comfortable position. Your head can hang down. On the inhale, raise your head and chest slightly while you alternate kicking your right leg and then your left leg straight back behind you, keeping your weight supported on your hands.

Hurdler.

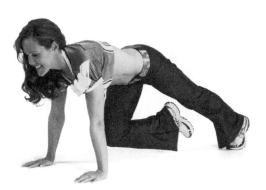 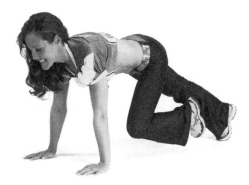

Pointers

As with the other Zone 3 exercises you shouldn't pause when you return your kicked back leg to the center. Keep a good steady pace.

HALFTIME BREAK: KICK SEQUENCE

Target: Cardiovascular exercise

Start: Stand with your feet comfortably apart and your hands on your hips, elbows bent.

Motion: Hop with feet together, then lift right knee; hop with feet together, then lift left knee; hop with feet together, lift right leg to kick waist height; hop with feet together, lift left leg to kick waist height.

Halftime kick sequence.

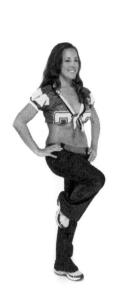
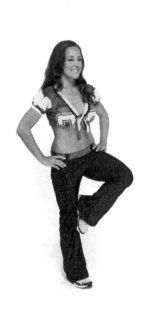
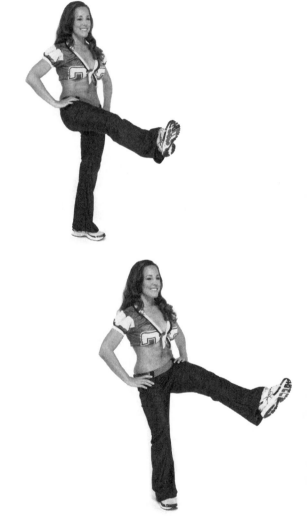

Pointers

Exhale every time you lift a leg! This is another rhythmic dance move, so stay in constant motion!

BLOCK 12

Zone 1: Plank Abductions

Target: Core (abs, pelvic floor, hips, and back), shoulders, back of arms, front of arms, outer thighs

Start: Lie in prone position (on stomach). Place your palms on the ground directly under your shoulders. Keep your arms and legs straight as you do a push-up. Pull your navel in so your body forms a straight line from the top of your head to your toes. Try not to let your hips flex. Push the ground away to fully support your upper body. Hold this position.

Motion: Slightly raise and abduct (move leg away from midline) and return to center one leg, then the other.

> ### Pointers
>
> Use the modified version in which you rest on your elbows instead of your hands if necessary.

Plank abductions.

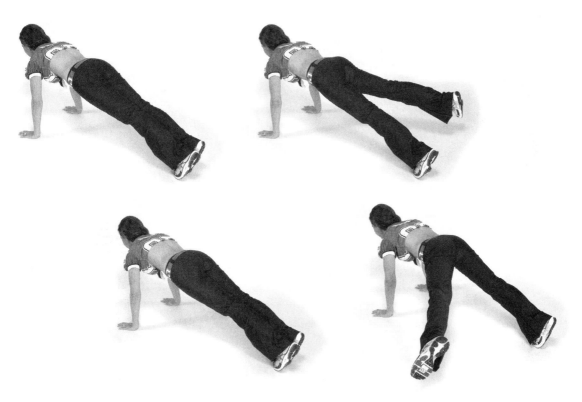

Zone 2: Warrior 3 Row

Target: Core (abs, pelvic floor, hips, and back), back of shoulders, upper back, back of legs, calves

Start: Hold one of your heavier weights in your right hand, with your arm hanging straight down. Begin in the Warrior 3 starting position: with hips and knees facing forward, arms to your sides, pivot your torso forward while you raise your right leg straight behind, eventually trying to raise to a position parallel to the ground. Do not flex your hips; hold your body in a straight line.

Motion: Pull the weight toward you so that your arm forms a 90-degree angle and your elbow is above your inclined body. Engage your upper back muscles as your elbow rises. Release your arm and return weight to the beginning hanging position, but do not lower your leg or change your position. Do ten repetitions. Switch legs and arms and repeat.

Warrior 3 row.

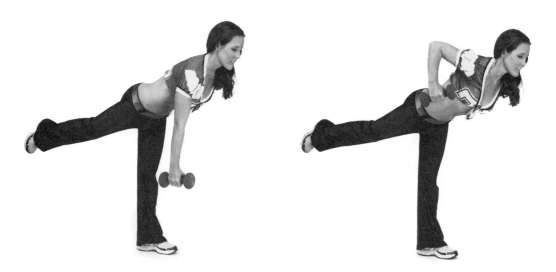

Pointers

Pull your navel toward your spine to work your abs and help you balance. Throughout the exercise, keep your arm tight to your body. If you find it impossible to stay balanced, place your free hand on your knee, and do not lift your leg (but do lean your torso forward).

Zone 3: High Knees

Target: Cardiovascular exercise

Start: Stand with feet six to twelve inches apart.

Motion: Run in place and lift your knees as high as you can. Pump with your arms. Imagine that you are running in knee-deep water and have to lift your feet out of it. Keep your chest and head high and your spine aligned.

High knees.

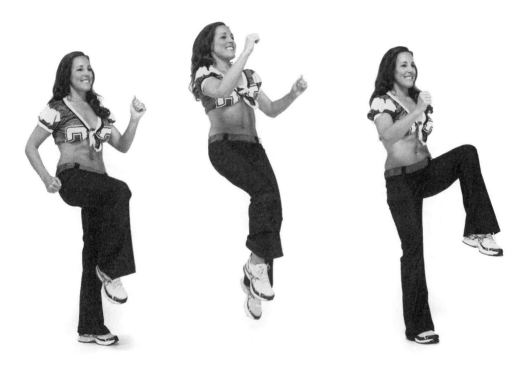

Pointers

Don't drop your head and chest. That will put too much strain on your lower back. Modify by simply lifting knees high, no running.

BLOCK 13

Zone 1: Game Clock

Target: Upper back, arms, butt, back of legs, front of legs, core (abs, pelvic floor, hips, and back)

Start: Get into the Warrior 3 starting position: with hips and knees facing forward, arms extended by your ears, lean forward on one leg, eventually trying to get the back leg parallel to the ground. Do not flex the hips. Hold your body in a straight line.

Motion: Move your arms away from your ears to your sides, pointing behind you, then back to the starting position. Do not release Warrior 3 until repetitions are completed. After ten repetitions, switch legs and repeat.

Game clock.

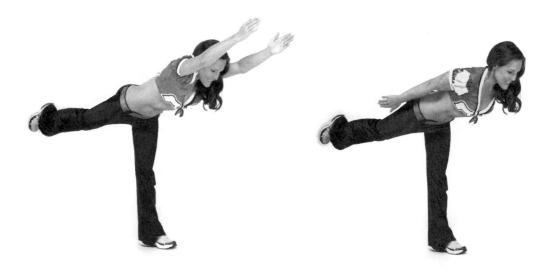

Pointers

Pull your navel in, and keep your shoulders and hips square to the floor. It is important to keep your arms by your ears. If you find this difficult when you are parallel to the ground, place your body on more of a diagonal.

Zone 2: Alternating Front Lunge with Core Isolation

Target: Legs, back of legs, inner thighs, outer thighs, calves, core (abs, pelvic floor, hips, and back), shoulders

Start: Stand with feet shoulder-width apart, arms extended overhead while holding one of your heavier weights with both hands.

Motion: Extend one leg in front of your body. Slightly flex your hips and knees to a 90-degree angle. Keep your weight centered. Straighten both knees and hips to upright position. Keep a neutral spine. Return to the starting position and step forward with other leg. Do not release your arms.

Alternating front lunge with core isolation.

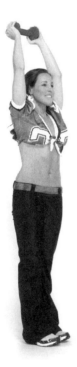 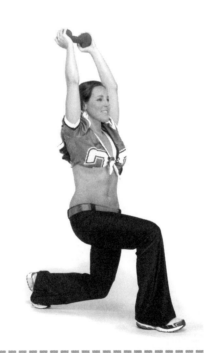

Pointers

Keep your knee behind your toe as you lunge forward, bend *both* knees, and keep your abs engaged.

Beginner modification: Eliminate the use of the weight.

Zone 3: Tackle

Target: Cardiovascular exercise

Start: Begin in a plank (push-up) position. Your hands should be slightly wider apart than your shoulders.

Motion: Jump both feet and knees forward so that you come into the frog position. Hop back and repeat.

Tackle.

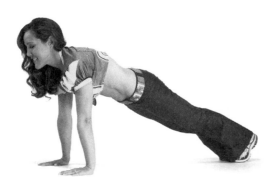
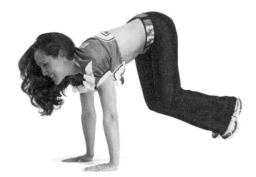

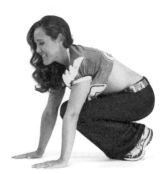

> ### Pointers
>
> As you bring your feet and knees forward, raise your chin and chest slightly. Don't rest in the frog position—immediately hop back and then forward again.
>
> Beginner modification: Perform the hurdler exercise from Block 11.

BLOCK 14

Zone 1: Push-up and Block

Target: Chest, shoulders, upper back, arms, core (abs, pelvic floor, hips, and back)

Start: Get into the modified side plank position: Kneel and place one hand to your side on the ground, arm fully extended to support you. Your other arm should be fully extended out and away from you. (Your body should form a diagonal line.) Concentrate on pushing out of the floor so you don't let your head sink into your shoulders. Try not to roll forward or back.

Motion: Drop your raised arm to the floor and roll forward into a push-up position. Perform push-up. (Keep your hands flat and head neutral. Your shoulders should be directly above your wrists. Keep those abs tightly tucked.) Extend into side plank on the other side.

Push-up and block.

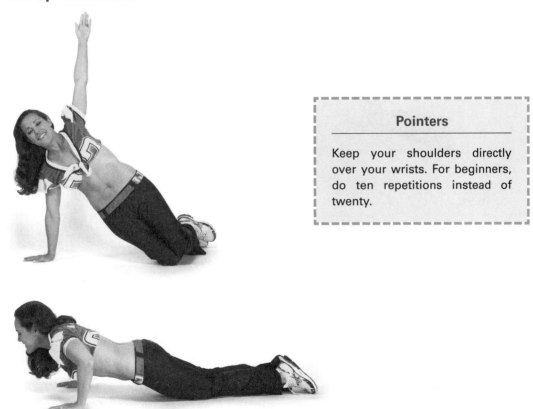

> ### Pointers
>
> Keep your shoulders directly over your wrists. For beginners, do ten repetitions instead of twenty.

Zone 2: Switch Lunge

Target: Front of legs, back of legs, heart

Start: Extend your right leg one to two feet in front of you and your left leg one to two feet behind you. Your heels should be raised slightly. Bend both knees and let the hips drop to the level of your knees.

Motion: Hop and bring your right leg back and your left leg forward.

Switch lunge.

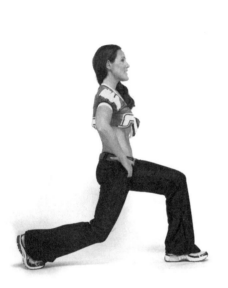

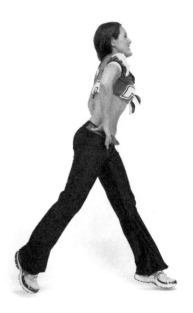

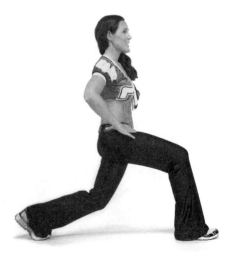

Pointers

Jumping as you switch your legs will provide a higher intensity.

Zone 3: Push and Press

Target: Cardiovascular exercise

Start: Begin on your knees in a push-up position. Place hands on a stair.

Motion: Perform a push-up on a stair, then push off the stair and lift your arms above your head. Modify this exercise by pushing off a sturdy wall or couch.

Push and press.

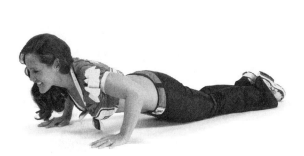
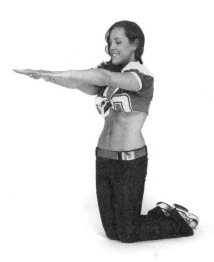

AB 5

Same as Phase 1 (series of five exercises—do twenty reps of each exercise). In Phase 2, challenge yourself by doing the advanced modifications included here.

Target: Core (abs, pelvic floor, hips, and back)
Start: Lying on your back, except for the back hyperextension, which you start by lying facedown.
Motion: See descriptions below.

Pointers

Keep your abs pulled in and down, so the lower back is anchored through all of these exercises. This is very important to make sure you are targeting the right muscles and to protect the lower back. Always breathe out on the exertion (raising yourself up) and breathe in on the rest (lowering yourself). Aim for twenty repetitions.

Elbow Tap

Sit on your "sitz" bones with your knees and hips flexed. Round your back and look at your navel. Extend both hands in front of you and pull back one elbow at a time so that it makes light contact with the floor. Hold your abs firm, and try to keep your legs and torso as still as possible. Advanced modification: Lean further back.

Elbow tap (Ab 5).

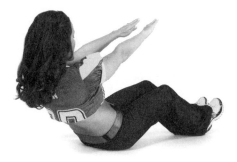

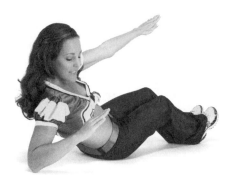

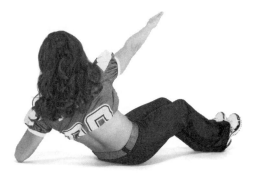

Scissor

Lie on your back and place your hands under your butt, palms down. While keeping your lower back on the floor, raise both your feet in the air above your hips with your legs straight. Lower one leg 45 degrees and bring back to center. Switch legs. Advanced modification: Lower the leg that is closer to the ground.

Scissor (Ab 5).

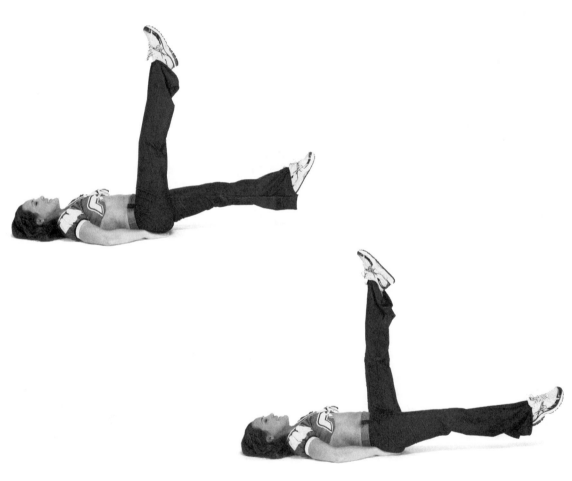

Scissor with Upper Body Twist

Lie on your back. While keeping your lower back on the floor, raise both of your feet in the air above your hips with your legs straight. Lower your right leg 45 degrees and twist your upper body to the left. Come back to center. Alternate legs. Lower your left leg 45 degrees and twist your upper body to the right. Interlock your hands behind your head and keep your elbows behind your ears while you twist. Beginner modification: Don't lower leg past 30 degrees from the floor. Advanced modification: Lower the leg as close as possible to the ground.

Scissor with upper body twist (Ab 5).

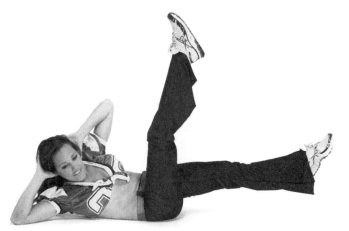

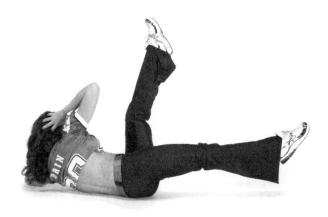

Bicycle

Lie on your back. Place your hands behind your head and keep your elbows back. Bring your right knee toward your chest and twist and raise your left shoulder up and toward your knee. Keep the left leg straight and held off the ground at a height according to your strength. The higher you hold the straight leg off the ground, the easier the exercise will be. Advanced modification: The lower you raise the straight leg, the more difficult it will be.

Bicycle (Ab 5).

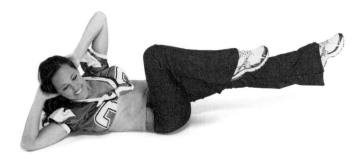

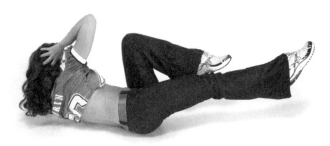

Back Hyperextension

Lie facedown with your arms extended forward, your elbows by your ears, and your feet together. Lift your upper body and lower body simultaneously. Lower yourself back to the starting position. Advanced modification: Lift higher.

Back hyperextension (Ab 5).

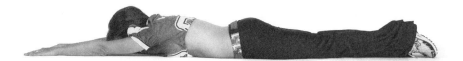

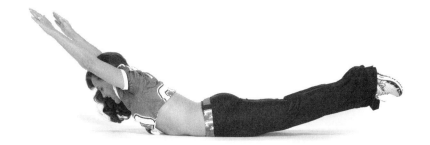

Week 5 (Monday, Wednesday, Friday)

Just as we did in Phase 1, we're going to eliminate one block and add another.

Do: Warm-up, Block 10, Block 11, Block 12, Halftime, Block 13, Block 14,
   Ab 5, Yoga Cooldown
Don't do: Block 9
Add: Block 15

BLOCK 15

Zone 1: Isometric Lunge with Woodchop

Target: Legs, shoulders, upper back, core (abs—specifically obliques—pelvic floor, hips, and back)

Start: You will need one of your lighter weights. Extend your right leg one to two feet in front of your body and extend your left leg the same distance behind your body, forming a triangle. Extend your arms fully in front of you at shoulder height. Slightly flex your hips and bend both knees to 90-degree angles.

Motion: Maintaining the lunge position, twist your core with your arms leading. Bring your hands to the outside of your right hip. Return your core and arms to the starting position without straightening your legs (hold the lunge). Pull your belly button in toward your spine. Be sure to switch legs and do twenty repetitions on the other side.

Isometric lunge with woodchop.

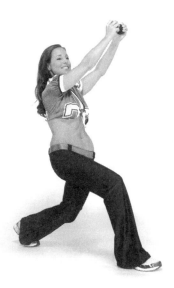 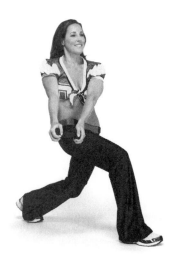

<table>
<tr><td colspan="1">Pointers</td></tr>
</table>

Pointers

Don't lock either knee, but keep your arms locked and straight.
   Beginner modification: Don't use the weight.

Zone 2: Grand Plié Sequence

Target: Outer thighs, inner thighs, butt, core (abs, pelvic floor, hips, and back)
Start: Stand with your legs two to three feet apart, toes pointed out.
Motion: Lunge with one leg (as you did above), rise, then lower into grand plié (push knees out). Lunge with your other leg, then rise and lower back to a grand plié.

Grand plié sequence.

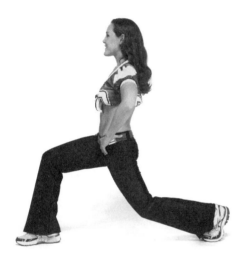
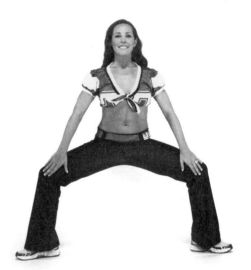
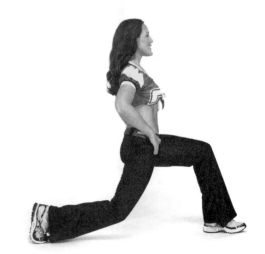

Pointers

Squeeze outer thighs during the plié—a li'l extra effort will make your buncakes burn!

Zone 3: Toe Touch

Target: Heart

Start: Stand with your feet together and your knees bent. Place your hands to your sides.

Motion: Jump and extend both legs to your sides (abduction).

Toe touch.

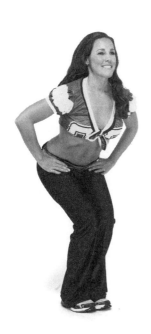

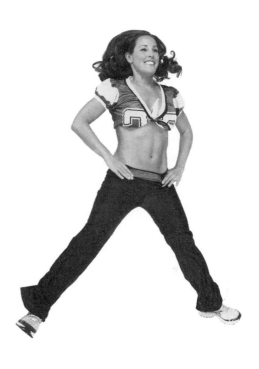

Pointers

Modify by performing a squat to leg abduction.

Week 6 (Monday, Wednesday, Friday)

Just as we did in Phase 1, we're going to eliminate one block and add another.

Do: Warm-up, Block 11, Block 12, Block 13, Halftime, Block 14, Block 15, Ab 5, Yoga Cooldown
Don't do: Block 10
Add: Block 16

BLOCK 16

Zone 1: Boomerang

Target: Core (abs—especially the obliques—pelvic floor, hips, and back)

Start: Get in the prone position. Place your elbows on the ground directly under your shoulders with your legs extended. Raise yourself so that your body is supported by your toes and elbows. Pull your navel in so you maintain a straight line from the top of the head to the toes. Hold this position.

Motion: Rotate and drop one hip toward the ground, then the other. Use the modified version (on your knees and elbows) if your back bothers you.

Boomerang.

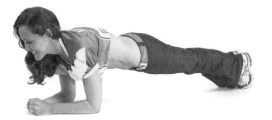

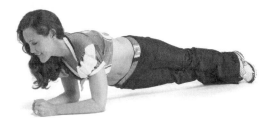

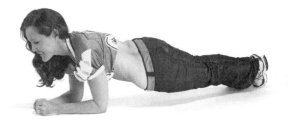

Zone 2: Lunge to Touchdown

Target: Outer thighs, butt, front of legs, calves, shoulders, core (abs, pelvic floor, hips, and back)

Start: You will need both of your heavier weights. Stand with your feet shoulder-width apart. Extend your arms overhead with one weight in each hand.

Motion: Step laterally with the right foot while keeping both toes pointing straight ahead. Bend your right knee to 90 degrees, keeping the knee behind your foot. Your left leg should stay straight. Simultaneously bring your hands on either side of your right leg. While pushing the right leg straight, raise the weights directly over your head with your palms facing forward. Switch legs.

Lunge to touchdown.

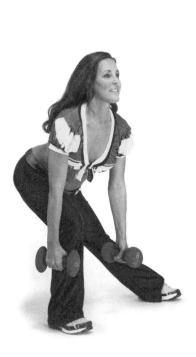
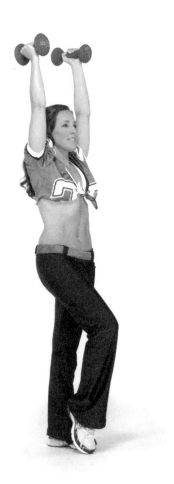

Zone 3: Jump Squat

Target: Cardiovascular exercise
Start: Stand with your feet shoulder-width apart. Place your hands on your hips.
Motion: Move into a shallow squat (so that your butt is at a 60-degree angle from the ground) and leap straight up.

Jump squat.

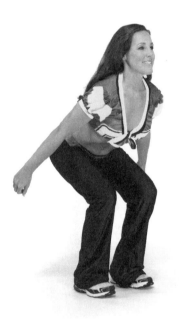
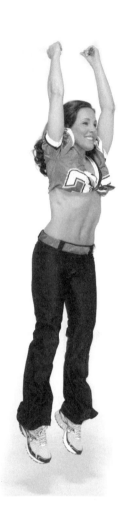

Pointers

Keep your chin up throughout the exercise. As soon as you land, jump again.

Cardio Workouts (Tuesday and Thursday)

Just as you did in Phase 1, in Phase 2 you will choose which aerobic/cardio activity to do on Tuesdays and Thursdays. Remember, because you are lighter and more fit, you will need to pick up the pace during these cardio workouts in Phase 2. Bump up the incline, bump up the resistance, or bump up the speed to get the most out of your cardio work.

THE 10-MINUTE WORKOUT

As in Phase 1, if you can't fit the usual Get into Your Fat-Burning Zone method into your schedule, spend one minute each on the following exercises:

1. Transverse crunch
2. Bridge knee abduction
3. Curtsy core isolation
4. Football push-up
5. Grand plié sequence
6. Football shuffle
7. Triceps dip
8. Woodchop to squat (right side)
9. Woodchop to squat (left side)
10. Ab 5 series

WE ALL NEED A LITTLE BOOST

Aimee is a member of the world-famous Los Angeles Lakers Laker Girl squad. Today she's a dancer and choreographer for a number of NFL teams. I spoke with her about her fitness and nutrition routines.

LB: Do you keep in shape by dancing? Or do you add fitness to your routine?

A: Dancing alone isn't enough. My body is used to it, since I have been doing it for so long. I had to incorporate core training and cardio to tone. I work out with a personal trainer two days a week.

We mix things up! Boxing one day, hiking sand dunes or working with the ball, resistance cords, and light free weights keep things fresh and exciting. I'm a petite person and I build muscle quickly, so toning is my main goal.

LB: What is it like to be a Laker Girl? Are you busy with media, charities, work, and games?

A: Being a Laker Girl is a full-time job with part-time pay and *a lot* of perks. Through being on the team, I was in movies, commercials, and TV specials and modeled for clothing lines and magazines. It was so much fun to do a little of everything! The team practices twice a week for three hours, volunteers for at least three charities a month, and dances at *every* home basketball game. That's almost sixty games a season, not counting play-offs. However, there are only a certain number of dancers on the floor at each game. So everyone gets about one game off per month. Promotional appearances generate the most money for the Laker Girls. However, the amount you are asked to do varies each month. It's very tough to have a full-time job on top of being a Laker Girl. Most girls are still in school, teach dance, or have a very flexible part-time job. Flexibility is key because on game days, the girls must be at the arena to rehearse by 3:00 or 4:00 p.m. Also, some promotional and charity events are scheduled on weekdays.

LB: You obviously have to keep up your energy. Do you watch what you eat to keep your energy high?

A: I believe in moderation. Portion size is *everything*! I eat what I want. But I try not to eat too much of it. So I eat small quantities multiple times a day to keep up my energy. Of course, I love fast food every once in a while. I just don't eat it all the time. But I would never deprive myself of anything I wanted to eat. Life's too short! I know when I die, I will never think, "I really wish I hadn't eaten that pizza and ranch dressing."

Aimee's workout routine incorporates a lot of variety, and that's what I've also done for you in Phases 1 and 2. Even though she's a dancer by profession, she has to do other things and raise her level of intensity to continue to see the benefits of all that work and play. I love Aimee's attitude toward food and eating, but notice that she does the exercise that lets her stay fit and eat what she wants!

Holly has been an Indianapolis Colts Cheerleader for the last five years. Even as a veteran cheerleader, she's still got amazing energy, owning her own business, running marathons, and generally keeping in shape. I asked her about her music motivation, and here's a list she gave me:

Kid Rock: "All Summer Long," "So Hott," "Roll On"
John Legend: "Save Room," "P.D.A."
Janet Jackson: "If," "Feedback"
Prince: "Kiss"
Maroon 5: "If I Never See Your Face Again," "Can't Stop"
T.I.: "Top Back," "Touchdown," "Show It to Me"
Trey Songz: "Can't Help but Wait"
Coldplay: "Trouble," "Viva la Vida"

H: Some of my other favorite artists include Corrine Bailey Rae, Lifehouse, Fergie, Madonna, Justin Timberlake, Chris Brown, and Britney Spears. And I'm a huge *American Idol* fan so I love music by these artists as well: David Cook, Chris Daughtry, Jordin Sparks, Carrie Underwood, and Kelly Clarkson.

If I am having a bad or "off" day, I find that if I exercise my mood will instantly change. Having an hour (or two) alone to clear your thoughts is instant therapy for me. I find running to be a very peaceful form of exercising. If I'm having an off day on game day I immediately surround myself with my friends on the dance team. We listen to music, dance, act silly, and tell funny stories that get us all laughing hysterically so that we are fired up and ready to dance once our feet hit the field. And as for me, smiling comes so naturally to me, especially once I'm on the field because I'm doing something I love to do . . . dancing and performing for our amazing fans!

I hope you can see that these are smart, fit, and fun women who are both serious about taking care of their bodies and dedicated to maintaining good health. But they also enjoy life and embrace it fully. They're able to find a balance between being alone and being with friends, working on their careers and caring for themselves. Not only do you need to work on your core muscles so that you can maintain your balance during your exercises, you need to work on your core self—family, friends, work, and leisure—to really get your life in shape.

MAINTAINING YOUR WEIGHT

I have a friend, I'll call her Jennifer, who was really into fitness. She was an athlete in college and a very good and competitive road runner after college. She tore her ACL (anterior cruciate ligament) in her right knee messing around playing basketball with her nieces and nephews. Following her surgery, she was very good about doing her physical therapy, but she couldn't run for six months. During those six months, she gained twelve pounds. That may not sound like a lot, but an additional twelve pounds on her five-foot-four frame had her feeling really pretty bad.

Jennifer could substitute some other exercises for her running, but she couldn't work out with the intensity that she was so used to. She loved to run and was used to being able to toss off seven-minute miles with no trouble. Well, postsurgery she was struggling to run ten-minute miles. Instead of running nearly fifty miles a week, she was only able to do fifteen to twenty. She started to really get down, feeling like she was never going to get back to being her old self again. I tried to tell her that it would just take time, but that didn't make her feel any better. "You know what really stinks? It was so easy for me to stay in shape, I never realized how hard it is to get into shape," she told me.

I asked Jennifer why that was, and she said, "When you're first getting into shape, it's really exciting. It's all so new. I remember the first time I was ever able to run five miles without stopping. It was thrilling! Now, anytime

I run, all I can think about is how I used to be able to do this so much faster and so much easier. It's just so hard to stay positive."

I'm sharing this story with you for several reasons. First, because during the writing of this book I gave birth. Life has a way of interrupting our other plans. Don't get me wrong, I'm thrilled to be a mother, but I also understand what my friend Jennifer was going through. It is mentally tough to get back to where you were before. I try to focus on the benefits of exercise and nutrition and realize that every step I take is getting me toward my goal, but it's still hard for a goal-oriented person to get back to the same place they were.

Second, life is always going to throw us curveballs—some we plan for, others we don't. The best-case scenario is that we plan for them, prepare ourselves mentally to get back to where we were in our fitness and nutrition game plan, and continue to progress.

If you've ever started on a fitness or weight loss program, you've probably experienced this already. One week you see really good and positive results; the next week you either lose a little or don't lose at all. You kick your workouts into a higher gear, get better about not nibbling between meals and snacks, and the weight comes off again. This on and off, up and down, roller-coasting, yo-yoing phenomenon is fairly typical. That doesn't make it any less frustrating, but it does mean that when you check into the Reality Hotel, some things are just going to be an expected part of life.

I know that can be discouraging. I know that sometimes life circumstances will change and it will be harder at certain times than others to maintain your nutritional and fitness discipline. What follows are strategies you can use to recover from those lapses and maintain your new and lower weight. Remember these basic principles?

Calories consumed = calories burned = weight maintenance
Calories burned > calories consumed = weight loss
Calories consumed > calories burned = weight gained

Well, they still apply. There's no getting around those facts, just as there is no getting around the fact that you will have to continue to challenge your fitness threshold. Before, it was enough to work your way through zones 1, 2, and 3. Now the challenge will be to stay in zones 2 and 3 when you work out. As a part of this maintenance chapter, I'll provide you with a new workout that you can mix in with your regular routines that will carry you over that threshold and help you maintain your weight. I'm also going to provide you with some meal plans that you can use when you notice that you've started to put on a few pounds.

When Is It Time to Gear Up?

Okay. We know that unless you are one of those extremely rare cases, you are going to need to gear up at some point to recover from a time when you just weren't able, for whatever reason, to keep with the program. Rule number one is this: Don't beat yourself up about it. It isn't healthy (unless you beat yourself up by kickboxing!), it does you no good, and when you feel bad about yourself it is way too easy to let things slip further. Don't go there! We all slip up a bit. The true test is what you do after those slipups occur to help your body recover from them. The sooner you begin the recovery the easier it will be. You should also take pride in being able to overcome those obstacles. You did it once, so you can do it again.

How do you know when you need to regroup and tackle your fitness a little harder? Once you've gotten to your target weight, do a weekly weigh-in. Keep track of this information in your food journal.

If you:	You should:
Lost weight	Add 1 starch, 1 dairy, 1 fat, and 1 protein to your weekly total. Continue to monitor your weight.
Gained two pounds	Go on high alert. If you haven't been tracking your consumption in your food journal, start to do so again. If you've been tracking it with the shortcut method, switch to the strict calorie-counting method.
Gained four pounds	Do two *additional* thirty-minute cardio workouts plus one high-intensity workout in this chapter.
Gained six or more pounds	Go back to Phase 2 of the fitness and nutrition plan. Recalculate your BMR based on your new weight.

Ideally, you will still be doing your workouts from the six-week plan. I can't emphasize enough the idea that you have to combine exercise and nutrition, especially when you are trying to maintain your weight loss. Neither nutritional modifications alone nor fitness alone will do the trick. Consistency is the key, and hopefully, once you've completed the Ultimate Six-Week Fitness Plan, you will *want* to keep working out.

Sample Maintenance Meal Plans

BREAKFAST
- ½ whole-wheat bagel with peanut butter = 1 starch, ½ protein, ½ fat
- English muffin with turkey bacon and two eggs = 1 starch, ½ protein
- Oatmeal and one apple = 1 starch, 1 fruit
- Small snack—eat protein and carbs to keep you full longer

LUNCH
- Out to lunch? Take half home for tomorrow.
- Grilled chicken sandwich, small green salad with oil-based dressing = 1 protein, 1 starch, 1 vegetable, 1 fat
- Whole-wheat pita with chicken, tuna, or turkey; cucumbers, tomatoes, lettuce, and peppers; and light dressing or mustard = 1 starch, 1 protein, 1 vegetable, 1 fat
- Large salad with light dressing (light on the cheese, eggs, and bacon—protein is calorie dense) = 2 vegetable, 1 dairy, 1–2 fat (from dressing)

SMALL SNACK

DINNER
- Grilled salmon, asparagus in olive oil, ½ baked potato = 1 protein, 2 vegetable, ½ starch, 1 fat
- Black beans and rice, served with a veggie (½ cup of each) = ½ protein, 2 starch, 1 vegetable
- Grilled chicken on a salad with dressing = 1 protein, 2 vegetable, 1 fat
- Pork chop, brown rice, small salad = 1 protein, 1 starch, 1 vegetable, 1 fat

- Stir-fry: two teaspoons olive oil; three ounces of any lean meat; peppers, tomatoes, green beans, squash, or any vegetables you like served over ½ cup brown rice = 1 fat, 1 protein, 1 starch, 1 vegetable
- Two beef fajitas with cheese and sour cream = 2 protein, 1 vegetable, 2 starch, 2 dairy, 1 fat
- One low-fat frozen dinner with a side of veggies = 1 protein, 1 vegetable, 1 starch

If you have followed the jump-start eating plan well and lost weight, you should be able to add 1 starch, 1 dairy, and ½ protein. That's a new reward for sticking with the plan and working so hard.

Lindsay's High-Intensity/Low-Maintenance Workout

To offset the effects of reaching a threshold and finding yourself on that plateau where your usual routine no longer has your weight stabilized, I've devised this routine that you can do three days a week every other day.

Once again you will be doing compound exercises (an exercise that works more than one muscle group *and* burns calories at the same time). As always you will use your core throughout the entire workout.

1. Warm-up
2. High-intensity Ab 5 (twenty reps each)
3. Main workout (twenty reps each)
4. Steps 2 and 3 repeated
5. Cardio component
6. Yoga cooldown and stretch

WARM-UP

Doing twelve repetitions of the Step Close, Step Open, Plank Walk, and Squat and Counterbalance amounts to about one minute each.

Step Close (12 repetitions)

Target: Front and back of legs (quadriceps and hamstrings)

Start: Stand with feet approximately shoulder-width apart and weight evenly distributed.

Motion: Take one small step forward with the left leg. Raise the right leg up to waist height. Grasp the right leg with both hands interlocking around your knee. Pull your knee in toward your chest. Hold for five seconds. Take three steps and repeat with left leg raised.

Step close.

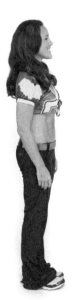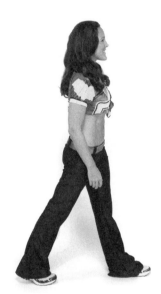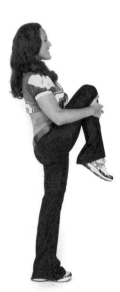

Pointers

As with all stretches, avoid quick bouncing movements. Work toward smooth, flowing movements. Concentrate on your breathing, exhale on the stretch, and hold your abs in to help you stay balanced on your one leg.

Step Open (12 repetitions)

Target: Front of leg (quadriceps), hips

Start: Stand with feet approximately shoulder-width apart and weight evenly distributed.

Motion: Take one small step forward with the left leg. With your heel leading, raise the right leg up and behind you. Grasp your ankle or top of your foot with the right hand. Gently pull the foot up toward your butt. When you feel a gentle stretch, hold for five seconds and then lower your foot. Take three steps and repeat with the left leg.

Step open.

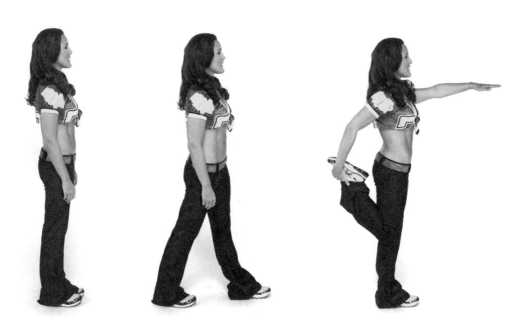

Pointers

When doing this or any stretching exercise avoid quick, bouncing movements. All of our stretches should involve long, smooth movements. Exhale as you stretch.

Plank Walk (12 repetitions)

Target: Arms, shoulders, back, core (abs, pelvic floor, hips, and back)

Start: Stand with feet approximately shoulder-width apart and weight evenly distributed.

Motion: From standing position, raise your hands over your head. Exhale and slowly bend at the waist until you are able to place your fingertips on the ground about twelve to eighteen inches in front of your feet and you can support your weight. Once you've balanced yourself on all fours, slowly walk your hands forward one at a time until your back is nearly parallel to the floor in push-up position. Hold for five seconds and walk hands backward toward your feet. Raise yourself up slowly to the upright position. For this raising motion, imagine that you are a rag doll or a puppet whose strings are slowly being pulled upright.

Plank walk.

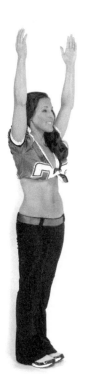
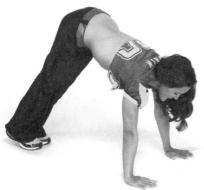

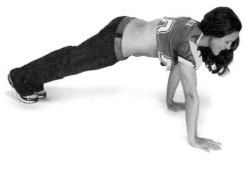
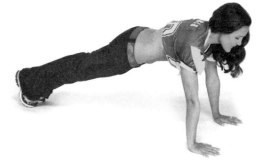

> ### Pointers
>
> If you have to bend your knees to achieve this position, do so, but don't squat down into a frog position. Try to keep your knees bent just slightly as you lower yourself.

Squat and Counterbalance (12 repetitions)

Target: Front of leg, back of leg

Start: Stand with feet approximately shoulder-width apart and weight evenly distributed.

Motion: On the exhale, simultaneously drop your butt and lower yourself into a squatting position until your thighs are parallel to the ground and raise your arms straight out in front of you. Keep your arms in front of you and hold for a five-count and then on the exhale gradually return to the starting position.

Squat and counterbalance.

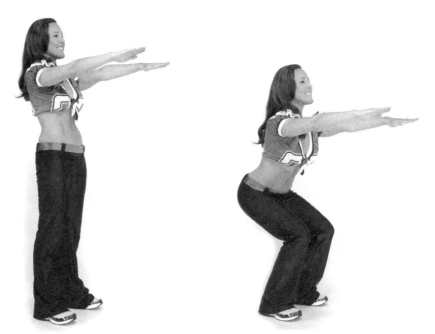

Pointers

Be sure to keep your chin raised and your eyes level throughout the exercise. Use your core muscles to help you lower and raise yourself in control. Going past parallel when squatting is not good on the knees, so stay parallel! To get used to how low to go, you can either do these in front of a mirror or have someone hold his or her hand at the back of your knees so that you just lightly touch it.

HIGH-INTENSITY AB 5—
A SEQUENCE OF PILATES CORE EXERCISES
THAT WILL FIRE THE AB MUSCLES FROM THE INSIDE OUT

Because you are now so much stronger than you were when you started, you can do this Ab 5 workout at the beginning without the risk of hurting those muscles.

For each, perform a set of 20, with no rest between exercises.

Back Hyperextension Twist

Lie on your stomach with your legs straight behind you. Place both hands behind your head and interlock your fingers. At the same time as you raise your legs off the ground, lift your head and chest from the floor. To add additional intensity to the exercise, rotate your arms and trunk so that you first tap your right elbow and then your left elbow on the ground.

Back hyperextension twist (high-intensity Ab 5).

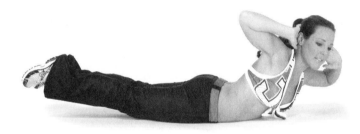

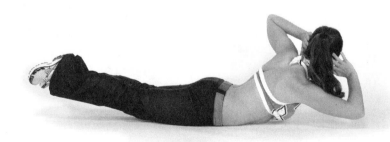

Plank Alternating Leg Lift

Place yourself in the push-up position with your arms straight and your elbows locked. Keep your back straight with your head in line with your spine and your core muscles engaged. Pull your navel in toward your spine. Raise your right leg behind you so that it is parallel to your back. Lower the leg and then raise your left leg to the same position. Everything but your raised leg should be still.

Plank alternating leg lift (high-intensity Ab 5).

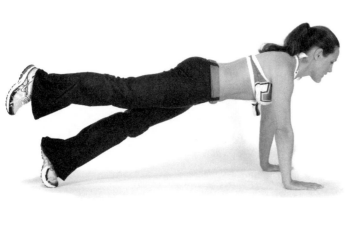

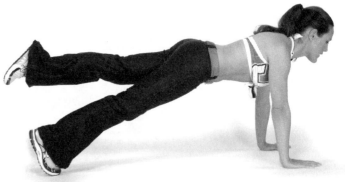

Knee Switches

Sit on the floor with your torso inclined as you rest on your elbows. Your legs should
be extended in front of you with your knees touching. Pull your closed knees
toward your butt and raise your heels slightly. Balance in this position for a count
of three. Next, rotate your legs from the hips to the right side. Keep the center
point of your body upright and pointed toward the ceiling. You should be pivot-
ing your legs around your waistline, while your torso remains still. Try to bring
your knees as close to the floor as you can without moving your torso. Return to
the center position and hold for a one-count. Twist to the left side as before.

Knee switches (high-intensity Ab 5).

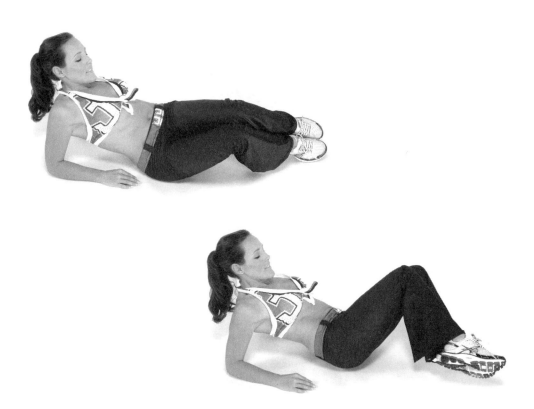

Bicycle

Lie on your back with your legs extended in front of you and your hands interlocked behind your head. As you slowly raise your head so that your shoulder blades are grazing the floor, lift your legs approximately six to twelve inches off the floor. Hold that position for a count of two. Pull your right leg toward your chest and bring your left elbow across your midline to touch your pulled-in knee. Push your right leg away from your chest and bring your left elbow back across your body past the starting point so that it touches the ground behind your head. Alternate legs.

Bicycle (high-intensity Ab 5).

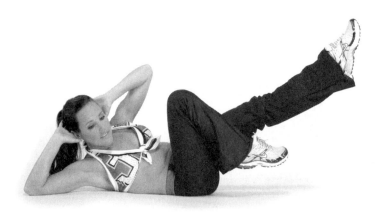

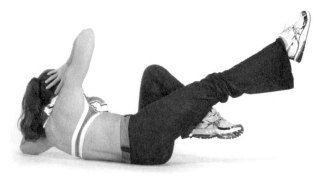

Pilates 20

Lie on your back with your arms extended along your sides. To begin the exercise, simultaneously roll your neck and shoulders off the floor while raising both legs. The lower you hold your legs, the more intense the workout. Maintain this position while raising both arms off the floor to a point just above your legs. Lower your arms while maintaining your body's position. Do not arch your back, and keep your navel tucked in toward your spine throughout the exercise.

Pilates 20 (high-intensity Ab 5).

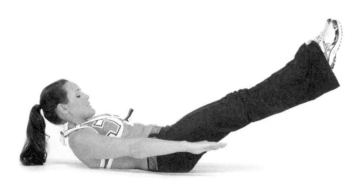

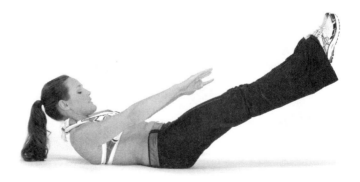

To refresh yourself on the basic forms of these exercises, refer to the descriptions in Phases 1 and 2.

Plié and Triceps Extension

With one of your heavier weights, plié and extend the arms as you straighten your legs.

Plié and triceps extension.

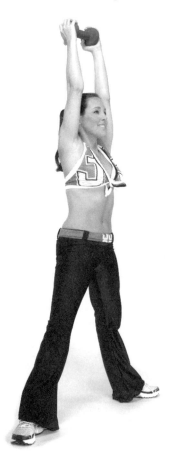
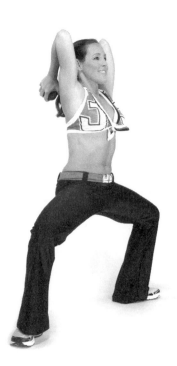

Stationary Lunge and Goalpost

With your pair of lighter weights, lunge and extend the arms overhead while straightening your legs. Keep feet stationary. Do twenty on right side then twenty on left side.

Stationary lunge and goalpost.

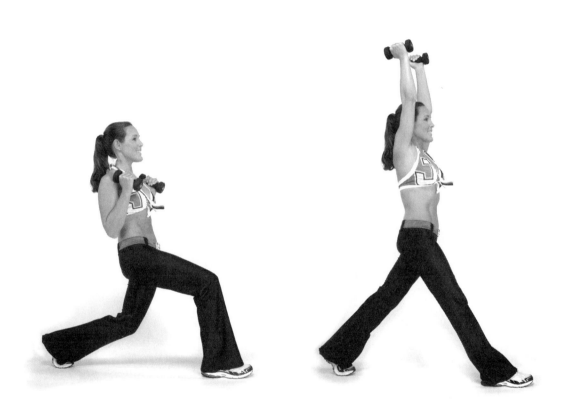

Plank Clock 3:00 and 9:00

From the plank position, move your right hand to the 3 o'clock position and the left hand to the 9 o'clock position. Return to starting position and repeat.

Plank 3:00 and 9:00.

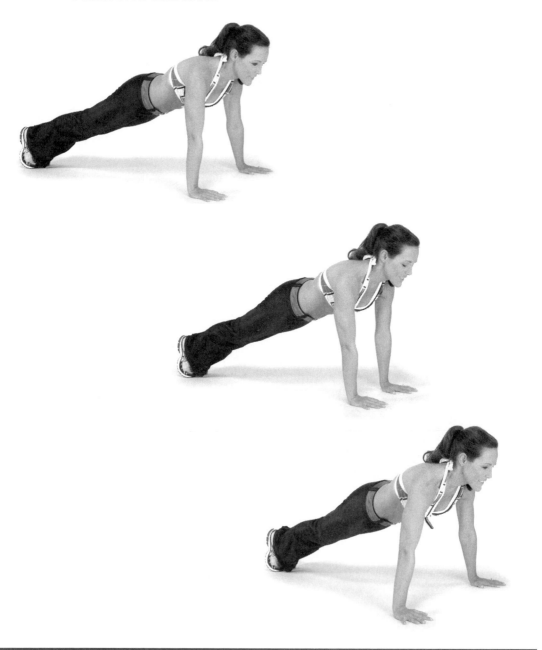

Squat and Kick

Hold your heavier weights down at your sides. Begin in the squat position, and as you stand each time, alternate kicking one leg in front of you. Bend your knee as you bring it up to kick.

Squat and kick.

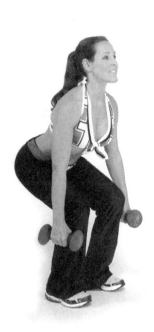
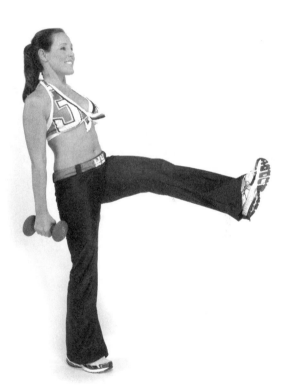

Plié and Lumberjack

Holding one of your heavier weights in both hands, plié and bring arms overhead. Remember not to swing the weight but to raise it in control using your muscles. Arms are straight throughout exercise.

Plié and lumberjack.

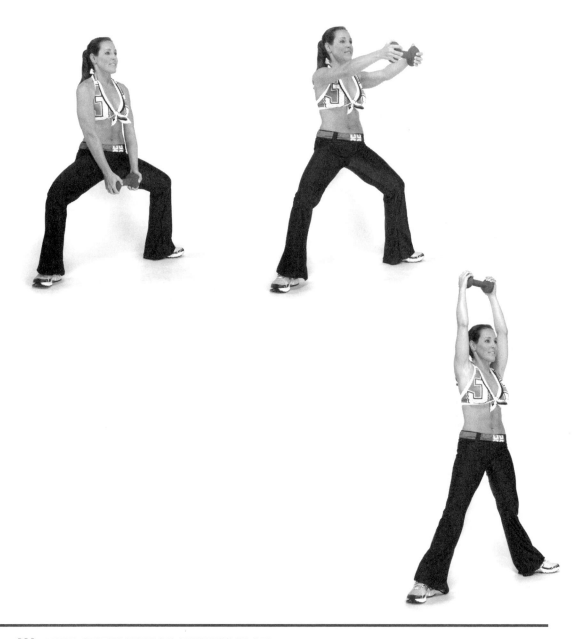

Biceps Curl with Core Balance

Using your heavier weights, perform this just as you did in Phase 1.

Biceps curl with core balance.

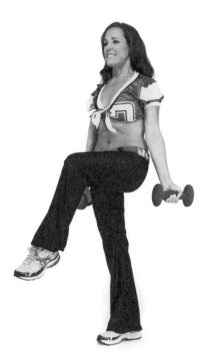 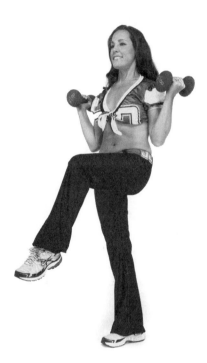

Squat and Abduct

Hold your heavier weights with each resting on a shoulder. Squat, then rise and lift your right leg to the side. Squat, then rise and lift your left leg to the side. Advanced modification: Perform twenty on the left, then twenty on the right.

Squat and abduct.

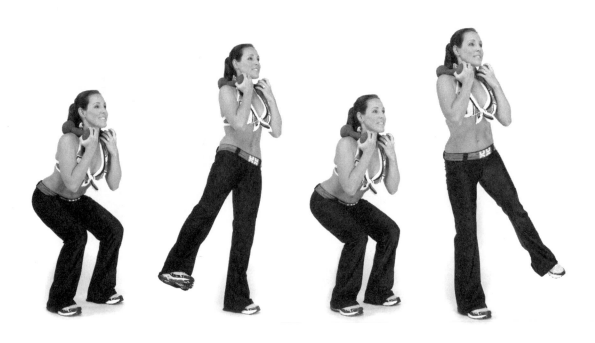

Plié and V

Hold your lighter weights down in front while you plié. Keep your arms straight as you rise and bring them up into the V. Modify by alternating arms instead of bringing them up simultaneously.

Plié and V.

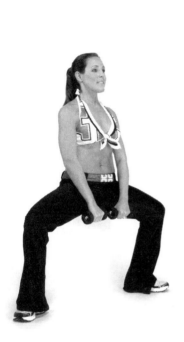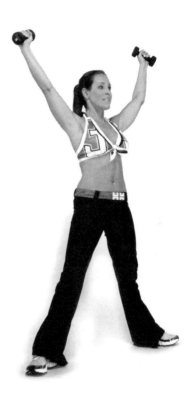

Eight-Count Push-up

Begin in the plank position. Drop your right knee to the floor and then drop your left knee to the floor. Do a push-up on your knees. When in the raised position, lift your right knee and then your left knee. Hold the plank position for two seconds before the next repetition. Do ten repetitions instead of twenty.

Eight-count push-up.

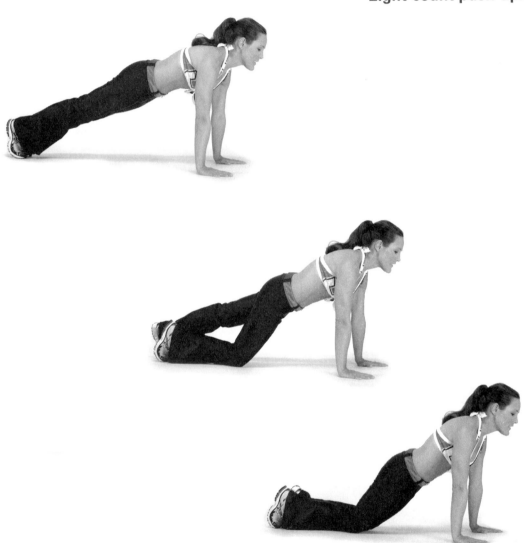

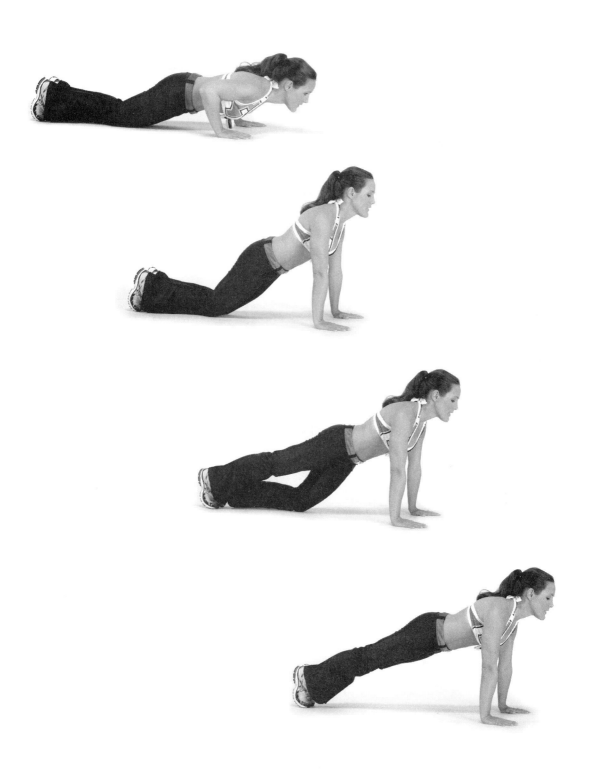

Grand Plié Sequence

With a pair of weights in your lowered arms, perform this sequence as you did in Phase 2. For greater intensity, use your heavier weights.

Grand plié sequence.

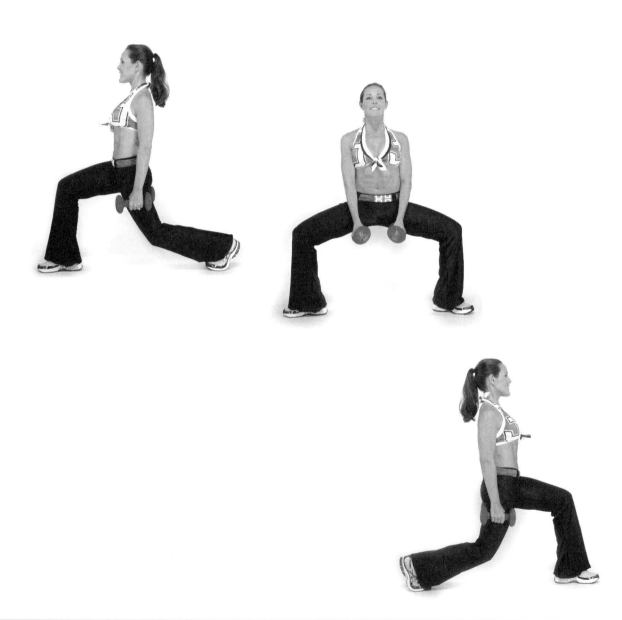

CARDIO COMPONENT

In Phases 1 and 2 of the Ultimate Six-Week Fitness Plan, you would have done a yoga cooldown at this point. Because I have to push you beyond your threshold, I'm adding a brief ten-minute cardio workout. I call this a cardio-climb, because instead of doing an interval with rests in between the sections of Zone 3 work, you will gradually increase the effort without the rests.

Do one of the following for ten minutes:

- Treadmill: Walk (at least four miles per hour), beginning with the incline at 1 and increasing it by 1 at one-minute intervals. Or jog at a pace of at least five miles per hour, beginning with the incline at 1 and increasing it by 1 at one-minute intervals.
- Elliptical: Begin with the resistance level at 1 and increase it by 1 at one-minute intervals.
- Bike: Begin with the resistance level at 1 and increase it by 1 at one-minute intervals.
- Running/walking outside: Find a hill and jog or walk it for ten minutes.

YOGA COOLDOWN AND STRETCH (SEE PAGE 250)

CARDIO MAKEUP DAYS

One way to "make up" for being bad—eating those extra slices of pizza, having a couple of drinks, or overindulging in any way, is to do an extra cardio workout to make up for it. If you are regularly doing your workouts, the day after your "bad" day, add an additional cardio workout to your routine. Here are some cardio workouts that incorporate interval training into them to maximize their effectiveness and to minimize the amount of time you spend.

Walk, Jog, or Run Outside: 30 minutes

Walking: Walk three minutes, jog two minutes. Repeat six times.
Jogging/running: Walk three minutes to warm up. Jog two minutes, run thirty seconds. Repeat jog/run ten times. Walk two minutes to cool down.

Treadmill: 30 minutes

Warm-up for two minutes.
Walk or jog with incline at 6 or 7 for three minutes; walk or jog with incline at 1 for one minute. Repeat seven times.

Elliptical: 30 minutes

Warm-up for five minutes.
Use a high resistance (all machines differ but shoot for 75 percent—i.e., 7 or 8 on a 10 scale) for three minutes then bring it down to 2 or 3 for two minutes. Repeat five times.

Kickboxing or Aerobics Class

You also can take a kickboxing or aerobics class on your makeup days.

Dance Jam, Core Metabolic Jumpstart, and *Shed 5 Fast* DVDs

I have DVDs available from my website, www.momsintofitness.com, which contain a variety of interval toning/cardio exercises. On your cardio makeup days, use the *Dance Jam* DVD. The *Dance Jam* is a fun, intense cardio workout without complicated hip-hop moves led by five NFL cheerleaders. And if you're looking for a variety of exercises to challenge your new body, try my other DVDs. *Core Metabolic Jumpstart* is an express core workout for the days you don't have much time. And *Shed 5 Fast* is just like our Ultimate Six-Week Fitness Plan with two thirty-minute fat-blasting intervals to choose from.

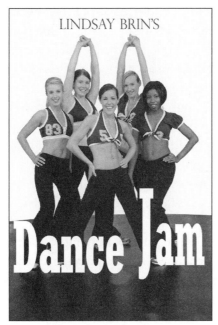

Dance Jam DVD.

Remember: Don't spend your time making up excuses; spend your time making up with cardio work!

~ 10 ~

YOGA: FABULOUSLY FLEXIBLE

Many of the cheerleaders I trained and cheered with had a background in dance. One of things we all recognized was that in addition to having cardio endurance, a good sense of rhythm, and a joy in movement, we had to be flexible. Many of the exercises I have included in the Ultimate Six-Week Fitness Plan are designed to improve your strength (tone) and work your cardiovascular system. They are also designed to get you moving and increase your flexibility. So far, I haven't said a whole lot about flexibility, how to develop it, and why it is important.

Flexible muscles are what most women idealize when they think of a toned, fit body. Most of us don't want bulging muscles, but we do want some definition or shape to our muscles. Long smooth lines are what we're looking for, and exercises like yoga target flexibility to help you shape and tone your muscles. Flexible muscles are less prone to injury and soreness. When you lengthen the muscle fibers (which is literally what you are doing when you are stretching and doing yoga), you are creating healthier tissue. If you've ever pulled (strained) a muscle, you know how sore you feel and how much that pain limits your range of motion and therefore your ability to move freely and easily. Have you ever had a muscle cramp? I'm talking about those really sharp, intense pains you get when your system is dehydrated (yes, that's usually the reason why you get a muscle cramp—drink more water!). Now imagine how much more intensely painful a muscle tear is.

When you tear a muscle, you literally shear the muscle fibers themselves, tearing them at a point near a joint where the tougher connective tissue (the tendon) joins the muscle to the bone. Muscle strains most commonly occur because of:

- Muscle tightness. Tight muscles are vulnerable to strain. Everyone should follow a year-round program of daily stretching exercises.
- Muscle imbalance. Because the quadriceps and hamstring muscles (the front and back of your legs) work together, if one is stronger than the other, the weaker muscle can become strained.
- Poor conditioning. If your muscles are weak, they are less able to cope with the stress of exercise and are more likely to be injured.
- Muscle fatigue. Fatigue reduces the energy-absorbing capabilities of muscle, making it more susceptible to injury.

That's why I have you do a warm-up and cooldown before and after every workout. Every NFL dancer I know and have worked with understands the importance of doing these pre- and postworkout routines. Yoga will help lengthen, loosen, strengthen, and balance your muscles. And by doing it at the end of your workout, it will help flush your system of the waste products that are produced when you exercise. Those waste products help contribute to you being sore. If you just stop working out and don't do a cooldown, you will wind up fatiguing those muscles. Yoga will help increase the blood flow to your muscles to not only flush out the bad stuff, but to carry nutrients necessary to repairing damaged muscle cells.

What Is Yoga?

Yoga literally means "union with yourself." It is a practice that has been around for thousands of years since it was developed in India. It has evolved and there are many different types of yoga, from Hatha, Vinyasa, Ashtanga, and Kundalini, to Bikram, Iyengar, and Pilates. What all of these have in common is an emphasis on the body and movement, and on the breath and the mind. Yoga is capable of helping you to relax, stretch, reduce stress and anger, heal, and gain personal understanding. That's a tall order for a fitness routine, but you have to remember that there is a very deep spiritual component to yoga.

I'm not going to spend time going into the deeper spiritual and philosophical elements of yoga, but for those of you who are interested, there are many resources available to explore the numerous facets of the practice. Instead, we're going to spend our time going through some of the basic principles of yoga practice and positions. Just like my Ultimate Six-Week Fitness Plan, the great thing about yoga is that you can enjoy its many benefits in a very short period of time. From the very beginning of yoga, its practitioners and those who helped it evolve were interested in efficiency. The relatively brief cooldown program I outline here isn't very different from the many classes and programs available to you. You don't have to dedicate your life to the practice to feel it working for you!

Yoga Breathing

We've already talked about diaphragmatic breathing and the importance of exhaling on the effort while doing the exercises. Yogic breathing shares some similarities with those concepts, but the major emphasis in yoga is concentrating on your breathing pattern as a way to eliminate many of the distractions of the outside world. Changing your breathing patterns helps to alter how you think—that's where many of the stress-relieving benefits kick in. Particularly since you'll be using this yoga workout as a cooldown, it will be important to begin this phase of the workout with some simple breathing exercises.

There are three purposes of these two minutes of breathing: slow down, detach, and focus. After the intense interval training you were doing, your heart rate and respirations rates will be elevated, so for the first two minutes of the cooldown, your priority is to get your breathing and heart rate back to, or close to, your resting rate. To help you both detach and focus, I recommend that you either stop using your music at this point or use songs that are far less up-tempo than what you use during the main part of the workout. Instead of trying to pump yourself up, you should be calming yourself down a bit. I also recommend that you use instrumental music. If you're anything like me, the lyrics of the songs will either be running through your mind or running through your mind and dancing across your lips. It's hard to detach and focus on what's going on inside you when you've got lyrics in there.

What you're focusing on, instead of the music you're hearing or any of the thousands of thoughts that are going to be cascading through your mind, is just your breathing. Yoga teachers often say, "Think of your breath breathing you, instead of you doing the breathing." That's a bit philosophical and kind of deep, especially since you don't have to think about breathing in order to breathe—you do it automatically. Instead, just closely observe your breathing and what it feels like when you breathe, how each of your muscles act. Here are some other helpful hints for yogic breathing:

1. Always breathe in and out through your nose. This is the opposite of what you were doing when breathing on the effort. When you breathe on the effort, you forcefully expel the air through your mouth.

2. Focus on the sound of your breath. If you close your throat just a bit, you'll hear a sound kind of like when you hold a jar to your ear. You'll also be able to feel the breath passing your throat and coming out cool through your nostrils.

3. If you are having trouble with hearing your breath, you can lightly cover your ears.

4. Close your eyes. Eliminating visual distractions will also help you focus.

5. Sit in a comfortable position. This should be a position you can hold for the two minutes of your breathing exercise. Keep your hips above your knees and your spine as straight as possible.

6. If you can't hold that seated position, you can lie down, but don't put a cushion under your head.

7. Keep your arms and hands relaxed but don't place them on your torso.

8. Don't hold your breath at any point.

The Breathing Techniques

These breathing exercises shouldn't take any longer than two minutes, and you should be able to move easily from one to the other.

ARCHED BREATHING

1. Get in your comfortable seated position.
2. Inhale through your nose and arch your back, bowing your chest forward, stretching your spine from its base to your neck.
3. Breathe out and curve your back in the opposite direction so that your shoulders are forward and from the waist up you form the letter C. Drop your chin slightly to complete the curve.

Repetitions: four

YOGIC DIAPHRAGMATIC BREATHING

Since you're already familiar with this technique, I won't go into any detail. For this part of the breathing exercise, simply stay in that comfortable seated position and do ten repetitions. What makes this yogic breathing is that you will inhale and exhale through your nose, and you will inhale and exhale for the same amount of time. Really concentrate on counting to at least four on the inhale and on the exhale cycle. The longer you can inhale and exhale the better, so if you can make it past a four-count, do so!

Repetitions: ten

STANDING EIGHT-COUNT BREATH

Rise from your seated position, while still doing the Yogic Diaphragmatic Breathing described above. With your feet comfortably apart, stretch your arms toward the ceiling and rise onto the balls of your feet and then gently lower yourself. Work toward inhaling to a count of eight and exhaling to a count of eight.

Repetitions: three

The Yoga Cooldown

This is the sequence of yoga positions you should do at the conclusion of every Get into Your Fat-Burning Zone workout. You will also be doing these yoga poses for Phases 1 and 2 and maintenance. These poses take years to master, so be patient.

Half-Moon pose.

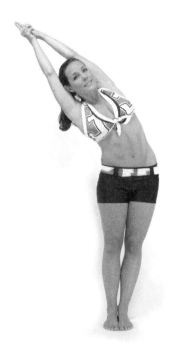

HALF-MOON POSE

1. Stand with your feet together and your toes spread slightly. (This is the standing start position, also known as Tadasana. For the other poses that begin this way, I will simply say get into Tadasana.)
2. Inhale and raise your arms overhead interlocking your fingers, but keeping your index fingers released.
3. Exhale and bend sideways from the hip so that your torso is directly over your right leg. Press your heels into the floor to stabilize your body. Keep your chest facing forward, stretching through the left side of your body. Inhale as you return to the center; exhale and repeat on the other side.

Repetitions: two on each side with an eight-count breath

Camel pose.

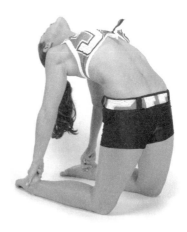

CAMEL POSE

1. Kneel on the floor with your knees as wide apart as your hips. Keep your back and upper legs straight by imagining that a wire is connecting the top of your head to a point directly above you on the ceiling. Keep your shins and tops of your feet pressed firmly into your mat.
2. Place your hands with your palms on the tops of your butt and point your fingers down. Push your tailbone forward toward your abs, but don't "pooch" out your stomach or your groin.
3. Inhale and raise your chest up and press your shoulder blades in toward your spine. Visualize your heart being lifted up and out toward the ceiling.
4. While keeping your head up, with your chin near your breastbone lower yourself backward so that your hands grasp your calves or feet simultaneously.
5. Please note: As a beginner, this is going to be hard, so if you can't achieve this position, you can lean your thighs back so that they aren't perpendicular (at a 90-degree angle) to the floor. You can also twist your torso to one side just a bit to get your hand on your calf or foot. Then return your torso to the straight position and place the other hand on that side's calf or foot.

Camel pose modified.

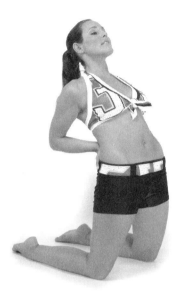

These pointers pick up from where we left off with the Camel pose.

6. Your lower ribs should be sticking out strongly toward the ceiling. If they are, raise your pelvis up.
7. The bones of your elbows should be facing straight back behind you. You can either keep your head in line with your spine or let it drop lower—but only if you don't feel any pain and you aren't straining the muscles in your throat.
8. Stay in this pose for two full eight-count breaths.
9. To get out of the pose, put your hands on the front of your hip bones. Inhale and lift your head and torso up while pushing your hips down toward the floor. Try to lead with your chest and not your head. Rest in Child's Pose for a few breaths (see page 267).

Repetitions: two

Warrior pose to Pyramid.

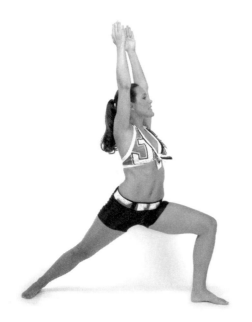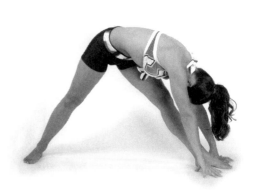

WARRIOR POSE TO PYRAMID

1. Begin in Tadasana.
2. Exhale and spread your feet greater than shoulder-width apart.
3. Angle your right foot in slightly to the inside and your left foot 90 degrees to the outside. Make sure your heels are aligned. Rotate your left thigh outward so that the center of your left kneecap is in line with the center of your left ankle. Inhale and stretch your arms above your head.
4. Exhale and bend your left knee over your left ankle. Your shin should be perpendicular to the floor. If possible, bring the left thigh parallel to the floor.
5. Stretch your arms so that they are parallel to the floor.
6. Turn your head to the left and look at your hand.
7. Hold for an eight-count breath. Then straighten your left leg and release upper body as you hinge at your hips. Lean over your straightened left leg. Hold for an eight-count breath.
8. Reverse your footing and repeat on the right side.

Repetitions: two

Cat-Cow pose.

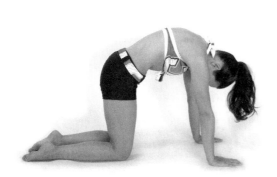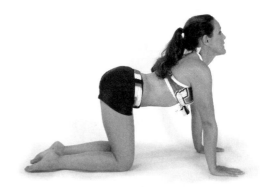

CAT-COW POSE

1. Begin on all fours, with your wrists in line with your shoulders and your knees in line with your hips.
2. Keep your spine, neck, and head all in a line. Visualize a line extending from your tailbone through the top of your head.
3. Exhale, let your belly drop, and slowly raise your chin toward the ceiling. This is the Cow pose.
4. Inhale, round your spine and drop your head, and look at your navel. Visualize a cat stretching in a Halloween decoration.
5. Repeat the Cat-Cow stretches: inhale for an eight-count into Cat and exhale for an eight-count into Cow.

Repetitions: two

Spinal twist.

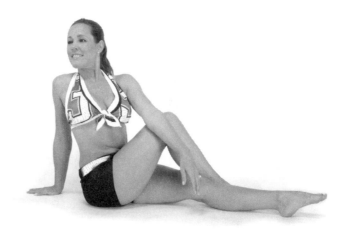

SPINAL TWIST

1. Sit on the floor with your legs extended straight in front of you.
2. Cross your right foot over your left leg and place it on the floor outside your left hip. Your right knee should point straight up.
3. Exhale and twist your torso toward the inside of your right thigh. Keep your right hand on the floor just behind your right butt cheek and press your left upper arm on the outside of your right thigh near your knee. Hug your chest to your inner thigh.
4. Keep your back straight and your head raised.
5. Continue to twist your torso to the right.
6. On each inhale lift your chest from your sternum, pressing up from the floor through your arm to help. Twist a little more with every exhalation.
7. Hold for two eight-count breaths, then release with an exhalation, return to the starting position, and repeat to the left for the same length of time.

Repetitions: two on each side

Pigeon pose.

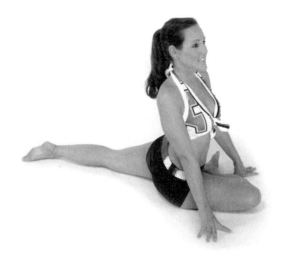

PIGEON POSE

Begin on all fours.

1. Pull your right leg up near your right hand.
2. Angle your right foot to the left.
3. Slowly extend your left leg back, and drop your pelvis.
4. Straighten your back as you push yourself above the extended left leg.
5. Support yourself with straight arms alongside the body, and sink even further down into the pose.

Repeat on other side.

Pigeon pose advanced.

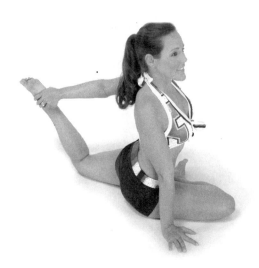

1. Square the hips toward the floor.
2. Place padding under the right side of your butt as necessary to bring the hips square or modify by bending the back leg.

Try the following variations:

3. Bring the torso down into a forward bend over the right leg.
4. Let the weight of your body rest on the right leg.
5. Continue squaring the hips and breathing into the tightness.
6. Make sure the top of the left foot keeps pressing down into the mat.
7. Come back up, bringing the hands in line with the hips.
8. Bend the left knee and reach back for the left foot with your left hand.
9. Draw the foot toward your butt, stretching the left thigh.
10. Square your shoulders to the front of the room.
11. Release the left foot, curl the left toes under and step back into Downward-Facing Dog (see page 261).
12. Repeat pose on the other side.

Staff pose.

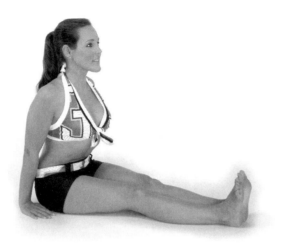

STAFF POSE*

1. Sit with your legs outstretched straight in front of you.
2. Clench your quadriceps and hamstrings while flexing your feet. You can raise your heels off the floor.
3. Sit as straight as possible. Again, visualize a wire going from the top of your head into the ceiling.
4. Make sure your shoulders are directly in line with your hips.
5. Get a deeper stretch in the hamstring by taking it into single-leg Staff. Inhale for eight, exhale as you lean over your leg for eight.

*This is also known as Dandasana: the basic starting position for seated poses.

Repetitions: two

Butterfly pose.

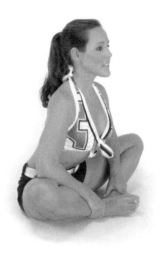

BUTTERFLY POSE

1. Start in the Dandasana seated position.
2. Bring your legs in toward your center so that the soles of your feet are together in front of you.
3. Grasp your toes and gently pull your heels in toward your groin.
4. While keeping your back straight, bend forward from the waist as you exhale.
5. Use your elbows to push down gently on your calves or inner thighs. Try to press them to the floor.
6. Release and repeat.

Repetitions: two

Upward-Facing Dog and Downward-Facing Dog.

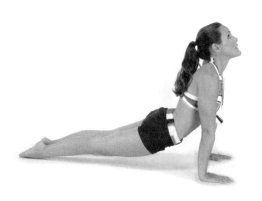 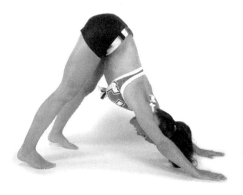

UPWARD-FACING DOG/DOWNWARD-FACING DOG

1. Lie flat on the floor with your hands next to your shoulders as they would be when you're about to do a push-up. Your toes should be in contact with the floor.
2. Come forward, rolling over the toes without letting your thighs contact the floor.
3. Press yourself up so that your arms are straight in the raised "push-up" position. Your chest should be perpendicular to the floor and your back in a hyperextended arch. Your body should be in the shape of the letter J, lying on its side.
4. Keep your legs engaged and off the floor, while pressing the tops of your feet down and dropping your hips.
5. Make sure you keep your shoulders over your wrists.
6. Transition into Downward-Facing Dog.
7. Lower yourself to the ground so that you're on your hands and knees with wrists aligned with your shoulders and the knees underneath the hips.
8. Curl your toes under and push yourself back with your arms while raising the hips and straightening your legs.
9. Rotate your upper arms outward to widen your collarbones and expand your chest.

10. Let your head hang, and prevent yourself from scrunching your shoulders around your ears by moving your shoulder blades away toward your hips.

11. Engage your quadriceps strongly to take the weight off the arms, making this a resting pose.

12. Rotate your thighs to the inside, keeping your butt high, and try to bring your heels flatly in contact with the floor.

13. As a beginner, it may not be possible to bring your heels down flat. Your muscles may still be too tight to accomplish this. Resist the temptation to walk your hands backward toward your feet to help bring your heels all the way down. Cheating like this won't help lengthen the muscles. Eventually you will be able to achieve this heels-flat position. Be patient. It will take some time for all the muscles to lengthen.

Runner's Lunge to Half Pyramid.

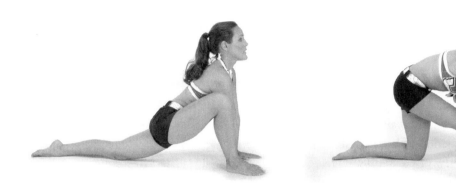

RUNNER'S LUNGE TO HALF PYRAMID

1. From the Downward-Facing Dog bring your right leg in front of you with the bent knee pointing up. Bring your hips down and place the top of your left foot on the ground with your left leg extended behind you.
2. Inhale for eight, then exhale for eight as you drop the hips.
3. As you inhale straighten your right leg and shift your weight to your left knee, so that it is now at a 90-degree bend. Exhale for eight.
4. Dancers: Drop the hips to the ground and lengthen both legs into the splits. This pose is optional—you can always repeat from the Runner's Lunge.

Repetitions: two on each side

That's it. Ten yoga poses that you can do in ten minutes. Optionally, you can end your yoga routine with Child's Pose (see page 267). I always find it a good way to relax and end my yoga time.

Incorporating yoga into your maintenance plan is a great way to continue to get the benefits of toning. While yoga isn't as intense of a cardio workout as some of the other exercises, you'll be surprised at how much it challenges your body in many ways. If you have achieved the goals you wanted to achieve through the six-week plan, then doing yoga a few times a week will really help you keep the weight off—if you continue to follow the nutrition plan, of course!

If you are still doing your fitness workouts, I suggest that you substitute yoga for one of your three fat-burning zone days. I really believe that the stress-reducing benefits of yoga will help rid you of some of the anxiety you may have surrounding your new nutrition and fitness lifestyle changes. So much of anything we do as humans is all about our mentality and being positive. I can think of no better way than doing yoga to help you feel good and look good!

Lindsay's Stress Less Yoga Workout

STANDING SUN POSE

Begin with your feet parallel and touching and your arms at your sides. Inhale and raise your arms straight away from you and then circle them above your head so that your palms are touching. Exhale as you bend forward from the waist, bringing your arms so that your head is between them. Keep your back as straight as possible for as long as you can. When you're bent as far as you can while still keeping your back straight, grab your ankles, calves, back of the knees, or wherever you can reach with both hands. You should exhale throughout this movement. Hold that grasping position for a few seconds without breathing in and then release your legs and slowly rise to the hands-over-head position while inhaling. Stretch and look at your hands above your head. Exhale and circle your arms and lower them to the sides.

Note: Extend your arms as far as you can throughout the circles to help expand your lungs and chest.

Repetitions: three

TWISTING TRIANGLE

This is a variation on toe touches. Spread your legs so that your feet are out past shoulder-width, but you don't feel any strain in the inside of your upper thigh or groin. Keep your toes pointed forward. Inhale and raise your arms and extend them outward at shoulder level. Exhale and bend at the waist, bringing your right arm across your body while raising your left arm straight up. Grasp the outside of your left ankle (calf, knee), and turn your head so that you are looking up at your left hand. Tug just a bit with your right hand to deepen the stretch. Hold for a count of two and then exhale and return to the starting position. Exhale and reach for the right leg with the left hand.

Repetitions: three on each side

TREE POSE

Start with your feet together and pointing forward. Stare at a point directly in front of you, keeping your chin level. Lift your left leg, and with your knee pointing slightly outward, rest your left foot on the inside of your right thigh, as high up on your thigh as it can go. Keep your toes pointed down and relax all the muscles in your raised leg to help maintain your balance. When you come to a comfortable balance point, slowly inhale and raise your arms straight above your head, bringing your palms together as you do so. While doing normal yogic breathing, count to at least ten and hold the position. Try to work toward being able to hold this position for a count of thirty. Don't tense your abs too much—that will restrict your breathing. Once you've held the position for a count of ten to thirty, slowly lower your arms and legs simultaneously. Alternate legs and repeat.

Repetitions: one on each side

ALTERNATE TOE TOUCH

Lie on your back with your legs together and outstretched and your arms over your head. Exhale completely and then inhale and raise your right arm and leg. Try to reach your toes without lifting your torso off the ground. Exhale and lower. Inhale and repeat with the left leg and arm.

Repetitions: three on each side

TORTOISE STRETCH

Sit with your legs in front of you and spread as wide as you possibly can without feeling a strain. Pull your toes back toward your body and support your weight on your arms held behind you with your fingertips pointed away from you. Raise your hips slightly and tilt your pelvis forward. Move your hands from behind you and gently rest them on your legs while you sit straight up. Imagine a line going from the top of your head straight up into the ceiling. Hold for a count of three. Return your hands behind you and repeat the movement two more times. Next, keeping your feet pulled back toward you, inhale and circle your arms over your head, bringing your palms together directly above you. Look at your hands and bend at the waist, angling toward your right leg. Grab your ankle (calf, knee) with both hands, and keeping your elbow bent, tug gently on your leg, bringing your upper body slowly toward your leg to deepen the stretch. Don't bounce! Smooth, slow, and steady movements are essential. Try to lower yourself to the point that you can grab your big toe and then work your way down to your arch. At this point, you should have exhaled completely. Hold for a count of two. Inhale and circle your arms over your head, look at your hands directly above you, and exhale while you circle your arms back to your sides. Repeat on the left side.

Repetitions: three on each side

TORTOISE STRETCH CONTINUED

Bend at the waist, bringing your head and chest directly in front of you as far as you can. If you can grab your toes, do so. Hold that position for a five-count and then slowly lift yourself back to the starting position. Remember to lead with your head and feel each separate vertebra folding as you move forward.

Repetitions: three

PLOW

Lie on your back with your feet twelve to eighteen inches from your butt. Bring your knees up to your chest and wrap your arms around them. Gently roll back and forth three times and then roll back a fourth time, bringing your knees to your forehead. Support your back with your hands on the back of your hips. Hold this position for a count of three. Exhale and extend your legs out behind you so that your toes touch the ground. Hold for a count of three. Relax your breath and bring your knees back to your forehead. Slowly roll forward until you come to a seated position.

CHILD'S POSE

Sit on your feet. Your knees should be together. Slowly bend forward until you can rest your forehead on the floor directly in front of you. Keep your arms at your sides and let them flop so that the tops of your arms from your fingertips to your elbows are resting on the floor. Settle into a comfortable position by wiggling. Focus on your breathing and relaxing all your muscles. Hold for at least a minute. If you can't get comfortable in this position, fold your arms in front of you and rest your head on your crossed arms.

I find the Child's Pose to be incredibly relaxing, and I can stay in that position for a lot longer than a minute! If you have any back or neck issues, I caution you to be extremely careful doing these yoga exercises. You should feel a stretch but not any sharp pains. I know a lot of people who have back trouble, and they do get immediate relief from going into the Child's Pose but you have to know your own body and be able to distinguish a slight discomfort from a stretch from real pain.

Ending with the Child's Pose should complete your stress less workout. Your heart rate and respirations should be back to normal resting rates, and you should feel really relaxed and content. Along with using this series of exercises as a cooldown, you can do them on days when you don't work out at all. If you come home from work and feel a bit stressed, take the fifteen minutes or so you will need to do these and feel the stress lifted. I have friends who suffer from headaches frequently, mostly because they carry a lot of their tension in their shoulders, and a quick yoga fix like I've described above does wonders for them.

You can also do the breathing exercises at any time. They are almost a form of meditation and when things get crazy at the office or at home, you can take a couple of minutes, shut your door, sit in a comfortable chair, and let a lot of your tension go, simply through breathing consciously.

STAYING MOTIVATED

If you need any additional motivation, know this: I'm going to be right there with you following this program. Twenty weeks after I gave birth to my daughter, Taylor, I got my body back. I wasn't exactly in the shape I wanted to be for this book's photo shoot, but I was almost there! Sure there were days I wanted to throw my hands up in the air, hand Taylor over to her grandmother, and curl up on the couch with some chips and dip in front of the TV. But was I going to hit my goal if I did that? I have to admit there was a day I did do that. And I also had my share of excuses: Should I work out or spend those thirty-five minutes writing my book? Should I spend the time on my website or just hang with my daughter? And what about sleep? But every time I gave into the excuses, all I felt was frustration and guilt when I woke up the next morning. My motivation was pure and simple—I wanted to feel good about myself again. And if I didn't feel good about myself, everything else would suffer (including my husband!).

So I woke up every day with a schedule. I made every effort to come close to checking off my to-do list. Many days I didn't even come close, but working out was at the top of my list so it got done most days.

In my effort to lose the baby weight, I had a little help at first with breastfeeding my daughter. It helped zap the weight off. But when she was about ten weeks old, I decided to stop and had to turn off the eating switch and get to it! When she was fourteen weeks old, we did the photo shoot for this book and I felt pretty darn good about my health. And when she was twenty weeks old, I had a better waistline than before!

We all need motivation. Yours might not be as simple as mine. You might need to pull out an old picture, your skinny jeans, or an ole friend. Whatever it is, find your motivation. I decided I'm going to give cheerleading another shot one of these days. Maybe some day you'll be flipping channels and see me on the screen cheering on the Rams. I hope you know that I'll be cheering you on, too.

CHEERLEADER BEAUTY TIPS

April, Oakland Raiderette—three-year veteran, mom to seven-year-old boy

- Get a good night's sleep before game day . . . it's important!
- Wear sun block with SPF 30. It's critical to protect your skin.
- Moderation is key when it comes to diet. Focus on eating fruits, vegetables, nuts, and lean meats. If I have a craving, I allow myself to have it instead of depriving myself. I believe that when you don't allow yourself to have certain foods, you want it more, which could lead to overindulgence.

Ashley, Houston Texans—three-year veteran, entrepreneur, cheer coach, fitness boot camp instructor

I've learned lots of beauty tips while cheering. I tell people all the time that cheering professionally has really helped me make the transition from girl to woman. There are so many tricks of the trade that pro cheerleaders use to achieve that flawless look. One of my favorites is the use of false lashes to get that starlike, eye-batting look. The lashes really help to open and enhance your eyes. Putting them on is another story, though. . . . Good luck!

Ashley, Houston Texans.

Aimee, Kansas City Chiefs and Los Angeles Lakers—three-year veteran; NFL and college dance team choreographer; business owner, Dance Team Designs

When you get so used to looking at yourself made up for games, you forget that game makeup is *not* everyday makeup. Remember you don't need a ton of makeup to look beautiful on a day-to-day basis. It's important to know the difference and see your game face as a costume. Don't walk around with heavy eye makeup and an inch layer of base and powder outside of games. It's terrible for your skin and it looks funny! Wear completely different makeup for games vs. everyday.

Erin, St. Louis Rams—three-year veteran, line captain, full-time student

I've learned tons of beauty tricks throughout the years through cheerleading, ballet, dance team, makeup artists, modeling experiences, and reading various magazines. Some of the ones I have learned through cheering are:

1. Putting concealer on your eyelids or a matte lid cream. MAC makes a great one—it will help keep eye shadow from bleeding and will maintain more intense colors longer.
2. Bronzers help minimize features, and light colors or illuminators help enhance features. For example, I have a very wide jawline and by putting some bronzer at the bottom of my jaw it helps to pull back this feature; putting some illuminating shimmer on the tops of cheekbones helps to highlight this feature.
3. When teasing hair, start with small, half-inch-thick strips that are parallel to your forehead, working from the forehead back to the crown of the head. Pull the hair forward, spray the roots with a hairspray or formula designed for the purpose of teasing (Helmet Head by Chi is my favorite), and using a bristle brush, gently pull the hair backward, teasing toward the root. Grab the next section and repeat. Lay the next section directly on top of the previously teased one, and when the brush grips the new section, it will grab some hair from the previously teased one, helping to blend the sections together, minimizing bumps. After all sections have been teased, flip hair back and brush according to desired style.

4. Keep your skin and lips hydrated!! This helps makeup and lipsticks to adhere more evenly.

5. If you know you are taking pictures, avoid foundations with SPF, as they can create a paler complexion in photos.

6. Use waterproof black eyeliner from Lancôme!

7. Lash primers work wonders underneath mascara.

8. When applying false eyelashes, wait until all other makeup is complete, then put a thin line of glue on the eyelash. Wait about thirty seconds to a minute to put the eyelash on. (Allowing the glue some time to dry ensures that it is already tacky for application and the lash will not slide around on your eyelid before the glue dries, messing up eyeshadow and gluing your eyelid together.)

9. Amazing way to shape eyebrows: Take a pen or pencil, hold it on either side of your nose. Your inner eyebrow should line up with it, not going past the side of your nose and the inside corner of your eye. Now line the pencil up with the outer corner of your eye and the bottom of your nose. The outside edge of your eyebrow should hit this point. The highest point of the arch of your eyebrow should be the outside of the iris, or colored part, of your eye.

10. If you would like a glimmer on your body or to define muscles, a small amount of baby oil gel can be used to create this sheen. (I learned this from my Pro Bowl friends who cheerlead outside in the sun, and from swimsuit calendar shoots.)

11. For a more natural shine on lips and not a glossy mess, put a dab of lipgloss in the middle of top and bottom lips over lipstick.

12. Makeup artist Barry once told me that eyebrows are the most important thing on the face, dominating the shape and how people perceive one's expressions. He said that one should never leave the house without groomed, defined (penciled or powdered in) eyebrows and mascara.

Brianna, Minnesota Vikings—two-year veteran, mother of a four-year-old girl and expecting baby #2, restaurant server, dance team coach

Oh, the secrets that I have learned! To give a few sacred secrets out . . .

1. To add a bunch of volume to any daily hairstyle (or evening glam) back-combing is amazing. I do it every day.
2. Pale skin is something in Minnesota we experience often, so the "Mystic Tan" or self-tanner is a huge help.
3. Washing my face every night and taking off all of the makeup and getting rid of all the dirt has given me great skin (also drinking lots of water).
4. Broadway nails are the best-kept secret of the MVC. They are the most natural-looking nails in the world. People will envy your nails with these on.
5. Smiling as much as possible and being around my amazing teammates gave me the best secret of all . . . being positive! That is contagious.

Tristina, Minnesota Vikings—two-year veteran, Pilates and yoga instructor, dance team coach

I put Vicks VapoRub on my lips every night before bed. It keeps them extremely soft and moist, especially through the Minnesota winters. The smell might be extreme at first, but once you try it, you will love it!

I also put mousse in my hair every time after I get out of the shower. I know it is a little '80s, but once you blow-dry it, the volume stays all day, and I always get compliments on how thick my hair looks.

Brooke, Arizona Cardinals—four-year veteran, real estate agent

When you are curling your eyelashes, heat up your eyelash curler for a few seconds with your blow-dryer before curling; it will have a curling iron effect. Also, when applying fake lashes, put the eyelash glue on the top of your hand first, then run the eyelash through the glue along the edge so you don't get too much glue on the lash. When you put it on your eye, start on the outside corner and press it toward the center.

Holly, Indianapolis Colts—five-year veteran, business owner

I am a firm believer that you need to take care of your skin as much as you need to exercise and eat right to stay healthy. I use a five-step skin care regimen on my face called Kara Vita. It includes a cleanser, pH-balancing mist, antioxidant, and SPF 15 face lotion. (The last two steps are a must to protect your skin from the sun's UV rays!) The entire product line takes care of fine lines, wrinkles, and dark circles. My favorite product is called Up Tight. It firms, lifts, and tightens your skin exactly where you need it!

Jennifer, Indianapolis Colts—six-year veteran, fitness professional, Indianapolis Colts Cheerleaders trainer

Keep a frequent workout program. It is healthy, increases your self-esteem, and gives you a great energy boost! You feel great!

A little tanning may be healthy . . . but too much is dangerous, ages the person, and it doesn't even look real or good.

Tryouts usually are in March and that means that I need to start getting mentally and physically ready in February (that means not a lot of "free time" in between seasons). In the past I made the mistake of following different diets, but after a couple of years I realized that for me, what works is watching my calories and balancing my diet and working out regularly with lots of cardio. Tryouts are tough because every year they expect more and more from you; in other words, if you are a vet, what you did last year is not enough, you have to step it up. So mentally I need to go with a very positive attitude and very focused on my goals (I know how fit I need to look to make it on the team). I also need to keep thinking of all the fun and excitement I can miss out on if I take anything in the process for granted.

Stacie, Kansas City Chiefs and San Diego Chargers—
three-year veteran; owner and creator, Zonas Designs
(the outfit I am wearing in the exercise pictures)

I feel that being an NFL cheerleader has taught me so much on beauty and a polished look that it literally has carried over into my everyday life. I always like to have a glow, so a self-tanner on the body and face is always helpful. Fake eyelashes are a must at promotions and game-day performances; they really open up your eye. I always use a lighter foundation under the eye to give the illusion of a "cat" eye. My cheerleader friends say Pureology has literally made their hair so much healthier and shiny, and has helped it grow. I combine that shampoo and conditioner with skin, nail, and hair vitamins. Since cheerleaders torture their hair with the curling iron and hairspray, it definitely needs as much conditioning and treatments to counteract and balance it out to stay healthy.

Tracee, Kansas City Chiefs—two-year veteran and two years working as game and practice coach, attorney

I learned during my time on the squad that one of the greatest inventions is spray tanning (you can go from white to beach-ready in less than a minute). Shading the abs and legs will make any imperfection easily concealable, sticky straps will keep any uniform piece in the right place with no wardrobe malfunctions, and high-lighter in the corners of the eye and under the eye will make you look as though you had a full eight hours of sleep even if you didn't.

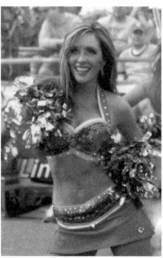

Tracee, Kansas City Chiefs.

Bethany, St. Louis Rams—three-year veteran, regional draught manager for a major brewery

The best beauty secret is the simplest of all. Drink lots of water. I still struggle with this one but it is so true. Getting the right amount of water does wonders for skin, hair, nails, and overall health.

Here are a few tips I learned from professional makeup artists during my time as a professional cheerleader:

- Runaway eyeliner: Apply your eyeliner to the top and lower lids. Then, using a small angled brow brush, dot the eyeliner line with black eyeshadow. This keeps your eyeliner from disappearing, running, or creating a black line in the crease of the eyelid.

- Corner eyelashes: It's not always necessary to use full eyelashes to create a more dramatic look. Use corner lashes or take a pair of lashes and cut them with scissors (in half or the corners) to get the lash look you want.
- Body bronzer: If you want a finished look with a soft glow, try using a loose powder with a light shimmer. Apply using a large powder brush to cheeks, shoulders, and stomach (if exposed).
- Lipstick color: Red is not the only color appropriate to wear with performance makeup. Use a color that is flattering and enhances your natural color and features.
- Clean face and clean brushes: Wash your face every night before bed. This removes oil, makeup, and dirt from the day and allows your skin to breathe. Also, wash your makeup brushes regularly. This extends the life of the brushes and makes it easier to apply makeup more evenly.

QUICK REFERENCE GUIDE

This is your quick reference guide for the Monday, Wednesday, and Friday workouts. For your cardio workouts on Tuesdays and Thursdays please refer to page 125 (Phase 1) or page 175 (Phase 2).

WEEK 1

BLOCK 1

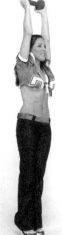

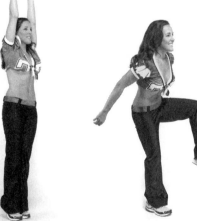

Transverse crunch.

Relevé and extend.

Yardline hop.

BLOCK 2

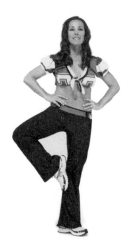

Plié to passé.

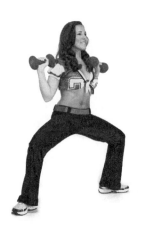

Lateral pulldown
and plié.

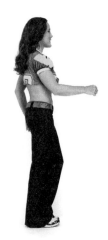

Stair climb.

BLOCK 3

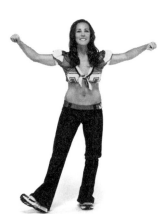

Heel jacks.

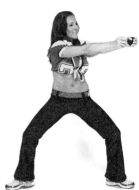

Plié and handoff.

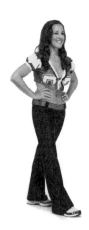

Ski.

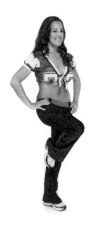

Halftime kick
sequence.

BLOCK 4

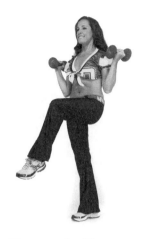

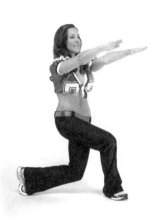

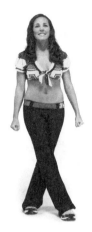

Biceps curl with core balance.

Curtsy core isolation.

Cross-jacks.

BLOCK 5

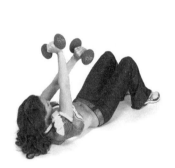

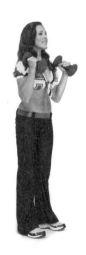

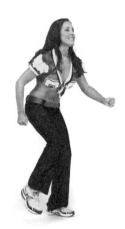

Chest press and crunch.

Goalpost squat.

Football shuffle.

BLOCK 6

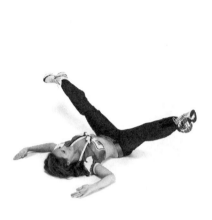

Inner-thigh adductions.

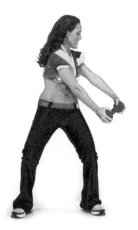

Woodchop to squat.

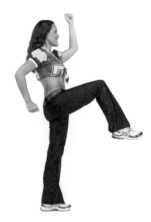

Bounder.

AB 5

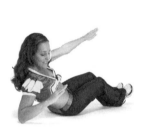

Elbow tap.

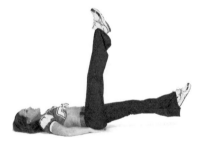

Scissor.

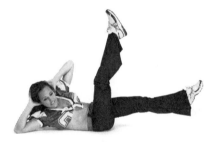

Scissor with upper body twist.

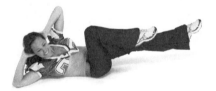

Bicycle.

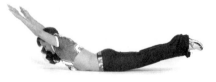

Back hyperextension.

YOGA COOLDOWN

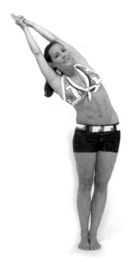

Half-Moon pose.

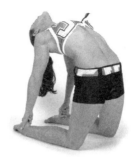

Camel pose.

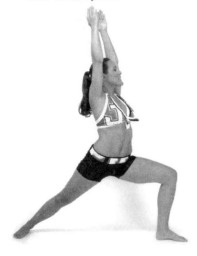

Warrior pose to Pyramid.

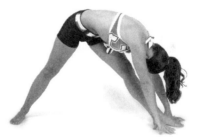

Cat-Cow pose.

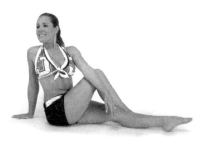

Spinal twist.

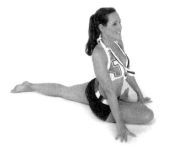

Pigeon pose.

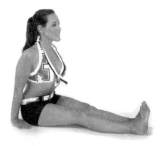

Staff pose.

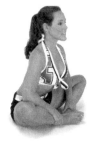

Butterfly pose.

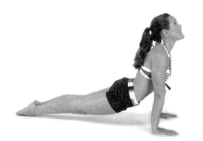

Upward-Facing Dog and Downward-Facing Dog.

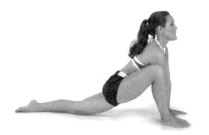
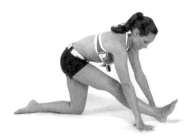

Runner's Lunge to Half Pyramid.

WEEK 2

Do: Warm-up, Block 2, Block 3, Block 4, Block 5, Block 6, Ab 5, Yoga
  Cooldown
Don't do: Block 1
Add: Block 7

BLOCK 7

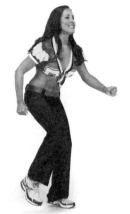

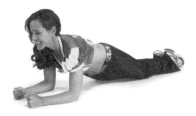

Modified boomerang.

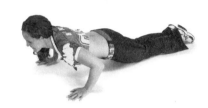

Football push-up.

Wide run.

WEEK 3

Do: Warm-up, Block 3, Block 4, Block 5, Block 6, Block 7, Ab 5, Yoga
  Cooldown
Don't do: Block 1, Block 2
Add: Block 8

BLOCK 8

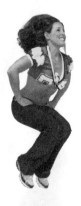

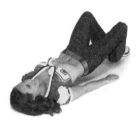

Bridge knee abduction.

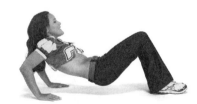

Triceps dip.

Plyometric tuck jump.

WEEK 4

BLOCK 9

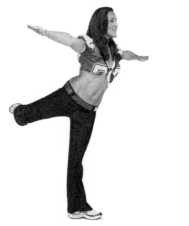

Chest fly and bridge.

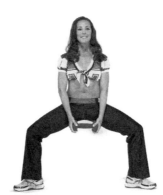

Mermaid.

Kick line.

BLOCK 10

Attitude lifts.

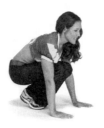

Plié and relevé.

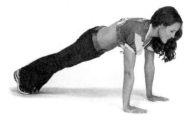

Squat thrust.

BLOCK 11

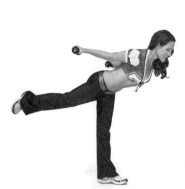

Triceps kickback in Extended Warrior.

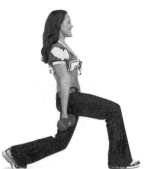

Reverse lunge to biceps curl.

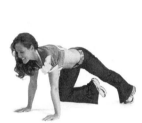

Hurdler.

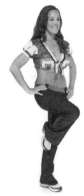

Halftime kick sequence.

BLOCK 12

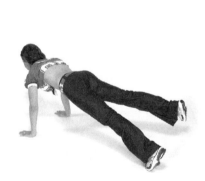

Plank abductions.

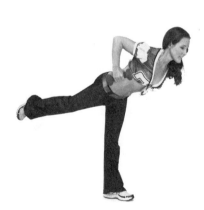

Warrior 3 row.

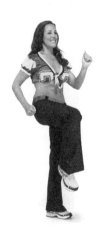

High knees.

BLOCK 13

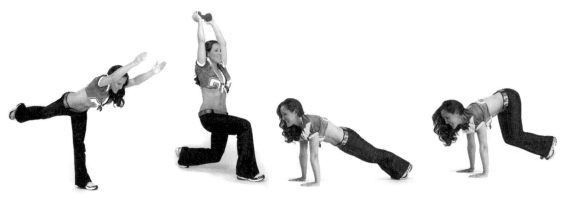

Game clock.

Alternating front lunge with core isolation.

Tackle.

BLOCK 14

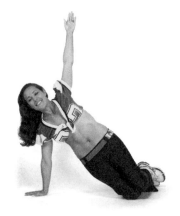

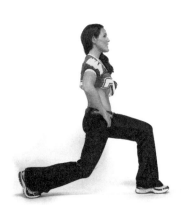

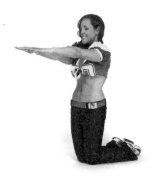

Push-up and block.

Switch lunge.

Push and press.

Repeat Ab 5 and Yoga Cooldown.

WEEK 5

Don't do: Block 9

Do: Warm-up, Block 10, Block 11, Block 12, Halftime, Block 13, Block 14, Ab 5, Yoga Cooldown

Add: Block 15

BLOCK 15

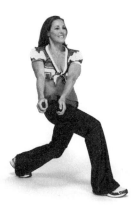 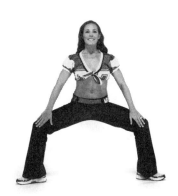 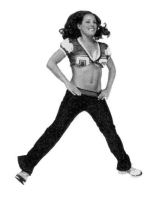

Isometric lunge with woodchop.

Grand plié sequence.

Toe touch.

WEEK 6

Don't do: Block 10

Do: Warm-up, Block 11, Block 12, Halftime, Block 13, Block 14, Block 15, Ab 5, Yoga Cooldown

Add: Block 16

BLOCK 16

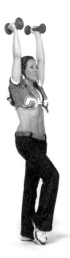 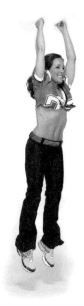

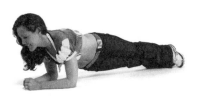

Boomerang.

Lunge to touchdown.

Jump squat.

THE CHEERLEADER FITNESS PLAN:
GOALS

_____

_____
_____
_____
_____
_____
_____
_____
_____
_____
_____
_____
_____
_____
_____
_____
_____
_____
_____
_____
_____
_____
_____
_____

· Food Journal ·

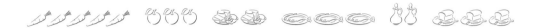

Breakfast: _____
_____
_____

Time:_____

Snack: _____
_____

Time:_____

Lunch: _____
_____
_____

Time:_____

Snack: _____
_____

Time:_____

Dinner: _____
_____
_____

Time:_____

• Food Journal •

Breakfast: _____

_____

_____

Time:_____

Snack: _____

_____

Time:_____

Lunch: _____

_____

_____

Time:_____

Snack: _____

_____

Time:_____

Dinner: _____

_____

_____

Time:_____

• Food Journal •

Breakfast: _____
_____
_____

Time:_____

Snack: _____
_____

Time:_____

Lunch: _____
_____
_____

Time:_____

Snack: _____
_____

Time:_____

Dinner: _____
_____
_____

Time:_____

• Food Journal •

Breakfast: _____
_____
_____

Time: _____

Snack: _____
_____

Time: _____

Lunch: _____
_____
_____

Time: _____

Snack: _____
_____

Time: _____

Dinner: _____
_____
_____

Time: _____

· Food Journal ·

Breakfast: _____
_____
_____

Time:_____

Snack: _____
_____

Time:_____

Lunch: _____
_____
_____

Time:_____

Snack: _____
_____

Time:_____

Dinner: _____
_____
_____

Time:_____

· Food Journal ·

Breakfast:_____
_____
_____

Time:_____

Snack:_____
_____

Time:_____

Lunch:_____
_____
_____

Time:_____

Snack:_____
_____

Time:_____

Dinner:_____
_____
_____

Time:_____

· Food Journal ·

Breakfast: _____
_____
_____

Time:_____

Snack: _____
_____

Time:_____

Lunch: _____
_____
_____

Time:_____

Snack: _____
_____

Time:_____

Dinner: _____
_____
_____

Time:_____

PHOTO CREDITS

With the exception of the images listed below, all photos
have been provided courtesy of Clyde Thomas Photography.

Tryouts, my second time around / *Lindsay Brin*
The swimsuit calendar shoot / *Lindsay Brin*
My official St. Louis Rams Cheerleader calendar photo / *St. Louis Rams*
The 2005–2006 Rams Cheerleader poster / *St. Louis Rams*
NFL Cheerleader calendar charity work / *Lindsay Brin*
Go, Defense! / *Lindsay Brin*
Girls from my line (and my husband) . . . / *Lindsay Brin*
The Calendar Reveal at our first game . . . / *Lindsay Brin*
My friend Erin and I in the locker room before a game . . . / *Lindsay Brin*
The St. Louis Rams Cheerleader dental sponsor / *Moms Into Fitness, Inc.*
My official Rams photo / *St. Louis Rams*
The swimsuit shoot / *Lindsay Brin*
One pound of lean muscle versus one pound of fatty tissue / *Lindsay Brin*
Dance Jam DVD / *Moms Into Fitness, Inc.*
Ashley . . . / *Houston Texans*
Tracee . . . / *Kansas City Chiefs*